A STRANGE PERIOD.

Insights into the Bizarre Experiences of Perimenopausal Women

by

Sheryl Gurrentz and Cindy Singer

o   o   o

iUniverse, Inc.
Bloomington

A STRANGE PERIOD.
Insights into the Bizarre Experiences of Perimenopausal Women

iUniverse books may be ordered through booksellers or by contacting:

iUniverse
1663 Liberty Drive
Bloomington, IN 47403
www.iuniverse.com
1-800-Authors (1-800-288-4677)

Cover by Cindy Singer and Sheryl Gurrentz

ISBN: 978-1-4620-7016-9 (sc)
ISBN: 978-1-4620-7019-0 (e)

Printed in the United States of America

iUniverse rev. date: 12/05/2011

Dedication

For all the women who have sweated it out in silence

and

For all the women who dared to bare their perimenopausal symptoms to their men, doctors, and/or non-perimenopausal friends and were told, "You're too young," "It's just your imagination," or, "You just need to eat healthier and exercise more."

and

For all our friends and family members who suffered through our incessant questioning about their perimenopausal experiences (in particular: Carol, Heidi, Sherri, Stacey, Robin, and especially our moms, Carol and Judith) and for Kim who shared her talent, creativity, and experiences so generously.

and

For all the women who will read this book and realize they are not alone, not imagining things, not going crazy, and should not be embarrassed to talk about (and laugh about) what they are experiencing.

Table of Contents

o o o

SECTION I

AND NOW, A WORD FROM OUR SPONSORS

WARNING: The content of this book is intended for hormonally-challenged women only and may be offensive and/or downright appalling to younger or male audiences.

READ AT YOUR OWN RISK!

Introduction: When Hairy Met Saggy

Have you been wondering if maybe you have early dementia, a thyroid problem, or some mysterious disorder that might explain some of the strange physical and mental changes you've been experiencing? If so, and you are in your 40's or 50's, there might be another explanation for your feelings: perimenopause. This stage of life, with all its confusing feelings and embarrassing bodily functions, is mysterious, frustrating, and long lasting. It deserves to be discussed even though it can be awkward to sit in the coffee shop with your girlfriends and have a conversation about topics such as vaginal dryness or hairy chins without attracting unwanted attention. Believe us, we have tried it! And, even if you are comfortable discussing it, your girlfriends might not be, even in private. Nevertheless, it is really important to know what other women have experienced. Then you'll know what's "normal," what's happening, and what's to come.

We certainly didn't set out to write a book about perimenopause. We just found ourselves gradually asking each other about changes we were feeling. First, it was strange periods. Then, it was odd hair growth, mental lapses, and unbelievable dryness. Overnight, it seemed we went from talking relentlessly about our children and every aspect of their lives to sharing the latest and greatest weird thing we were experiencing. As we did when we were pregnant, when we had little kids, and when we were preparing to write our previous books, we decided to do some research to get expert opinions. Much to our surprise and chagrin, there was not much there. We found many books written by doctors (most with pictures of women our mothers' ages on the covers). We looked, we really did, but we just couldn't find anything that felt practical and supportive, not just informative. We wanted to hear about the personal impact of perimenopause, not just the physical effects. We wanted accurate information about how to live our lives during perimenopause, not just about hormones or alternative treatments.

When we didn't find helpful, non-medical, non-hormone-related resources for women our age, we started talking about our experiences even more. We quickly began seeing the humor in our misery and the sheer joy and relief of sharing it with someone else. We got some of what we needed when we talked to each other and friends. There were many times when we would start discussing it with an unsuspecting victim and, before you knew it, she began spilling her hormonal guts about what she was experiencing — purging the secrets that had been building up inside and elated with relief that she was not the only one. We felt bad for the women who were clearly experiencing many of the same things we were, but just weren't comfortable having conversations about the gory details that we were becoming comfortable discussing.

One evening, after a margarita and lots of conversation about our most recent physical discoveries and our frustration with the lack of appropriate information to help us cope, one of us yelled out, "We should soooo write a book!" Like all ideas while intoxicated, we decided it was nothing short of brilliant! At first it was just something to laugh about, but then, as we realized we were experiencing more and more strange symptoms and still not finding the information we craved, we started seriously considering the idea.

Clearly, there was a need for a resource that targets our age group, talks about more than hormones and hair loss, and shares many, many women's stories as well as offers practical, helpful information. We can all agree there seems to be a lack of clear information about what the stages of "the change" are and that there is very little information on how many of us are experiencing perimenopause or menopause. There is definitely an inaccurate presumption that those of us who need this type of information are in our late 50's or 60's. While some of us certainly are, many, many of us are not.

We decided we needed to take matters into our own hands. We needed to encourage women like us to start talking about their experiences regardless of age and stop letting anyone dictate what is or isn't accepted as part of the perimenopause process. We also decided that if no one else can provide the resources we need, we would.

You will read about many of our own experiences in this book. To protect the innocent, namely our partners and completely mortified teen-aged children, we have not disclosed which stories are ours, however! We have also gathered and shared stories from women of various ages and stages of perimenopause at real and online "Hormonal Happy Hours." The result is hundreds of short musings that are easy to read (especially when you are having trouble seeing or concentrating). They will show you that:

You are not alone, not imaging things, and not going crazy!

There are some stories that have helpful information. Others will make you giggle. A few will give you the guilty pleasure of knowing you are not the only person who felt a certain way. There are also "What to Try" sections that offer multiple suggestions for making things better. The technical aspects of perimenopause are important, but they are not the focus of this book. There are plenty of other resources for that.

Our goal is to help you know that your experiences during this strange period of life are normal and, when taken with a grain of salt (preferably around the rim of a margarita glass when you're out with your girlfriends), worthy of a good laugh. This is not about figuring out the "best" way to deal with the time when your hormones are fluctuating as you approach menopause. It is about embracing, exploring, understanding, commiserating, sharing, and especially laughing! We'll talk frankly and honestly about the subtle and not-so-subtle experiences that comprise the journey from regular periods to anything but regular periods, to the end of periods. Period! We want to be like your best friends, telling you secrets that no one else will share with you, giving you permission to acknowledge your own frustrations, and supporting you through every bizarre experience no matter how strange this period of life gets. Read on, girlfriend!

Chapter 1
WTF?? – Defining Perimenopause

Dear Mother Nature: Today I called my BFF and screamed, "My vagina is a stranger!" I don't get it I've spent my whole life with her, we go everywhere together. Now, you have switched her with this dried up, unpredictable, alien vagina. WTF??

And, it is not just my vagina. It's so much more. Is there a word or phrase that could be used as a catch-all to refer to all of those things that make us women and make us different from men? You know, those thoughts and feelings that are known only to women? That voice inside, the fears, hopes, and worries that only women know? Whatever that word would be, that is the part of me that all of a sudden feels so unfamiliar. Why do I feel so different?

So what is the best way to describe this strange period we are going through? We already used the term perimenopause, but is that the right word? There are so many different terms being used out there. Let's make sure we can accurately describe this oh-so-special time in women's lives, identify what it involves, and define how long it will last. We will start with some very reliable resources.

First, we'll check out "premenopause" on Merriam Webster's Dictionary Web site. Premenopause is defined as, "the premenopausal period of a woman's life, especially perimenopause." Helpful, not! Let's try "perimenopause." Slightly more helpful: "The period around the onset of menopause that is often marked by various physical signs (such as hot flashes and irregular periods)." OK, plan B ... Dictionary.com. "The period leading up to the menopause during which some of the symptoms associated with menopause may be experienced." Hmmm. Don't worry, ladies. We will not give up! We have a 40-pound American Heritage dictionary on the desk that has never failed us. "Premenopause: of or relating to the stage of life immediately before the onset of menopause." Duh! Let's try "perimenopause." Nothing! LOL. It figures.

OK, now we're getting somewhere. The following definitions are from the Web site of the Women's Health division of the U.S. Department of Health and Human Services:

Premature Menopause: When menopause happens before age 40, it is considered early. Early menopause can be caused by certain medical treatments, or it can just happen on its own.

Perimenopause: Perimenopause, or the menopausal transition, is the time leading up to a woman's last period. Periods can stop and then start again, so you are in perimenopause until a year has passed since you've had a period. During perimenopause a woman will have changes in her levels of estrogen (ES-truh-jin) and progesterone (proh-JES-tuh-RONE), two female hormones made in the ovaries. These changes may lead to symptoms like hot flashes. Some symptoms can last for months or years after a woman's period stops.

Menopause: Menopause is the point in time when a woman's menstrual periods stop. Menopause happens because the ovaries stop producing the hormones estrogen and progesterone. Once you have gone through menopause, you can't get pregnant anymore. Some people call the years leading up to a woman's last period menopause, but that time actually is the menopausal transition, or perimenopause (PER-ee-MEN-oh-pawz).

Helpful, but it sort of leaves us wondering how long we will experience symptoms before actually hitting menopause. This website also states that the average age when women experience menopause is 51, but it can happen anywhere from age 40 to 55. So, you may ask, why do all the books, magazines, ads and TV programs show women in their 60's and 70's as "menopausal" and experiencing all the lovely symptoms we are going through right now in our 40's or early 50's?

Misery loves company, if the saying is right. Do we even know how many of us are currently experiencing perimenopause? Nope. Interestingly enough, if you go to government Web sites, you will find statistics on things like fertility, death, and kidney transplants. You will even find statistics on interesting topics such as pertussis and frequency of restaurant meals. But you won't find statistics on perimenopause or menopause. You will find 47 million hits on Google™ for "prostate" but only about 1.4 million for "perimenopause" and 30 million for "menopause." There are about 7 million hits for "hysterectomy" even though far fewer women have hysterectomies than go through perimenopause. Maybe we should just be content with having far more resources for conditions that (1) involve men and/or (2) can be measured by doctors, than for conditions that involve natural fluctuations that about half the adult population experiences.

Since there is no one clear indicator that a woman is in perimenopause, apparently there is no way to measure how many women are in this stage of life. However, there are some fairly impressive deductions that we can make from the statistics that do exist. According to the US Census Bureau, the two largest age groups of women, by far, are 35-44 and 45-54. From this we can deduce that the vast majority of females in this country are about to, are in the process of, or are just finishing perimenopause.

Most of us started to have periods when we were in our early teens. We can expect to stop menstruating at about 50 or so. Given that our life expectancy is approximately 78, we will likely spend half our lives with periods and/or estrogen production and half without. Is it any wonder that it takes a while to pass from one stage of life to the other? This is a major transition!

Just for fun, here is another interesting/frustrating tidbit: when you look for statistics on perimenopause and menopause on the U.S. Department of Health and Human Services Web site for The Office of Women's Health, you will find more information on prostate cancer trends than on trends in perimenopause. Hmmm. Does that mean that tracking our male partners' cancer is more informative about our health as women than our own hormonal changes? But, we digress. Deep breath... Back to the point...

Okay, let's assume that we sort of understand the time line. We can also assume there are an awful lot of us feeling the same way mentally and physically. Just like during puberty and pregnancy, perimenopause is a time of great hormonal change. Everyone agrees with that. There is no way to predict from day to day, let alone month-to-month or year-to-year, how we will be affected.

Since the existing resources don't seem to agree on what happens when and don't provide any specific information about how you'll know you are in perimenopause other than vague references to hot flashes and irregular periods, again we will provide our own kind of measuring stick to help determine whether or not you're perimenopausal. PS: If you don't "get" some aspects of the following definition, be very grateful!

You Know You Are Perimenopausal When:

♀ The only other viable alternatives are that you are pregnant, going through a second puberty, and/or have very early onset Alzheimer's.

♀ The phrase, "I laughed so hard I almost wet my pants" turns into, "I laughed so hard I wet my pants" — and you didn't laugh all that hard.

♀ You talk about your hairy asshole and you are not referring to your husband.

♀ You can start using the old saying, "not by the hair of my chinny chin chin."

♀ You have, at least once, seriously considered completely stripping off every single piece of your clothing in a public place in order to cool down.

and/or

♀ You have half the energy and need twice the exercise.

♀ You have to eat half as much, but have twice the appetite and gain twice as much.

♀ You have half the hair on your head, but twice the hair on the rest of your body.

♀ You have half the sex drive just when it takes your guy twice as long.

♀ You have half the periods, but they are twice as bothersome and you spend twice the time worrying about them.

♀ You have half the bladder volume and need to make twice as many trips to the bathroom (and have half the amount of time to get there once you feel the urge).

No matter what each woman's personal experience is, it is time for these lovely, oh-so-glamorous experiences to be brought into the light, where women can face them together. There may not be ways to control everything that is going on with our bodies, but we will do the best we can to get through it with grace and humor!

Now that we know what this period of life is called and have a preview of some of the effects, let's really delve into what we can expect of our minds, bodies, souls, sex-lives, and relationships over the next few years.

o   o   o

○   ○   ○

SECTION II

THEY JUST DON'T MAKE 'EM LIKE THEY USED TO!

At our most recent birthday lunch (a long-lasting tradition to celebrate our birthdays that are days apart), we had a long gripe-fest about how practically everything in our lives seemed to be breaking down. A washing machine should last more than 9 years, shouldn't it? Why is that horrible sound coming from under the hood of a car with 80,000 miles on it? Is it unreasonable to expect bedroom furniture to last longer than 15 years? Shouldn't all the burners on a stove be expected to heat identical pots of soup in the same amount of time when you are expecting 25 people over for a holiday dinner?

Why is a well-cared-for body that is only 40- or 50-something years old suddenly taking much longer to recover from a late night, becoming increasingly unpredictable with respect to menstruation, and failing to respond to the same makeup, hair, and exercise strategies that have worked for so long? We realized that we were starting to sound like our grandparents: Things just don't last like they used to! It's a pain to replace our appliances, cars, and furniture, but with the right amount of time and money, it can be done. Not so with our bodies, of course.

Accepting that we are old enough to have furniture that is a couple of decades old and children who are old enough to be in college or even have their own children (whether or not we actually have these things) is an important aspect of liking your body, even when it isn't looking or feeling like you want it to. Fighting the aging process is only going to waste your time. We recommend embracing it and making the most of it. Now, this doesn't mean that you shouldn't whine about the bodily changes that you are experiencing. We think that talking about your body and what it's doing to you is actually downright necessary. That's what girlfriends are for! In fact, the times when we share our latest disgusting experience, admit what is scaring us, and commiserate over the latest wrinkles can actually feel like therapy.

Seeing your body from a different perspective can also be really helpful at this stage of life. Go look at a picture of yourself from 10 or 15 years ago. Do you like what you see? Do you think to yourself, "I actually looked good! Why didn't I appreciate my body more back then? I actually could have gotten away with wearing shorts, but I thought my thighs were too fat!"

Now, project yourself 10 or 15 years in the future. Short of plastic surgery and participating in a reality TV weight loss show, things aren't likely to look much better than they do now. We bet you'll look back at pictures of yourself now and think that today's body is pretty damn good. Despite what you are going to read about in the next few chapters, try as best as you can to appreciate what you've got, even if your perimenopausal body is driving you crazy.

This is a great time to invest in yourself. Identify the things you like about your body and flaunt them. Do what you have to do to hide the wrinkles, excess flesh, dry skin, weight, or anything else you don't like — hopefully without obsessing about them. Invest in your well being, whether that involves medical care, natural remedies, or other third-party assistance such as facials and waxing. Buy the products you need, such as vaginal lubricant and reading glasses, even if it embarrasses you at the check-out counter. Celebrate who you are now so you don't have to wait another decade or so to like the body you have right now.

Chapter 2

Par for the Course – *Expected* Physical Changes

Dear Mother Nature: I guess that if you can give a big dose of hormones at puberty and turn a little girl into a lovely young woman, I shouldn't be so surprised that you can take them away and turn a lovely, 40-something year old woman into a droopy, drippy, dry, dumpy, ditzy one.

Are we "in" menopause, "going through" menopause, "in" perimenopause, "premenopausal" or what? Is menopause what you are in when your periods have totally stopped or is that post-menopause? We originally thought women first had irregular periods, then started having the expected menopause symptoms like hot flashes, weight gain, and trouble sleeping once they stopped having periods. Now we know, however, that the worst symptoms can actually be during the time when your hormones are fluctuating before your periods have stopped. Does that mean that once the hormones have leveled out at their new levels, these symptoms will go away or will there be different ones?

Although we asked and addressed some of these same questions in the first section, we are repeating them again on purpose. It is so important to understand that you are not alone if you are partially or even totally confused about what is happening now and what might happen in the upcoming years. There is good reason for the confusion.

It is shocking how many articles, from very credible sources, say that menopause is when your periods have stopped and perimenopause or premenopause is the time when your hormones are fluctuating in the years before your periods totally stop. Then, the very same article will go on to talk about the symptoms of menopause including irregular periods. Huh?

Then, there are other resources that say perimenopause includes the year after your last period. And still others say the year after the last period is actually menopause itself, which means that by the time you know for sure that you are in menopause, you are really post-menopausal. Some say that menopause is the point when you have gone 12 months with no period. This would mean, presumably, that menopause is the split second that is exactly 12 months after your very last period ended.

No wonder we are confused. No wonder many of us thought we would get symptoms like hot flashes and irregular periods while we were in menopause instead of the years leading up to it. The experts themselves seem confused and unable to communicate what they mean in an effective way. Clearly, there are some perimenopausal symptoms that continue once you are in menopause or post-menopausal, but the resources aren't very clear about what to expect there, either. So, we are left to discuss amongst ourselves what we are experiencing and hope that the experts eventually catch up.

In the Heat of the Moment: Hot Flashes /Night Sweats

Remember when a flasher was a creepy, naked guy in a trench coat? Now it is a 40/50-something-ish woman who can go from 98.6 degrees to the temperature of the surface of the sun in 98.6 nanoseconds.

Hot flashes are the "poster child" symptom for perimenopause. As common as they may seem, they are also tricky and unpredictable little bastards. They sneak up on you, they come and go at will, they get you at the worst possible times, and they never happen when you are freezing cold and would welcome one. They are also different in frequency and intensity for every woman. If you can't relate to the following stories from the women we've talked to, count yourself as one lucky sister!

♀ I wake up regularly in the night with a pool of sweat on my chest between my breasts and my hair soaking wet at the base of my neck. It's disgusting.

♀ I don't get many hot flashes, but I definitely get night sweats. I now put a towel down under me and an extra t-shirt next to the bed. When I get wet, I can just change my shirt and take the towel out from under me.

♀ Why do we have hot flashes during the day and night sweats at night? Aren't they the same thing?

♀ I have a high powered fan and a space heater under my desk at work, and on a typical day, both get used multiple times.

♀ Hot flash is the wrong label for what I experience. Flaming inferno would be more appropriate. I am not just hot; I am on fire internally. I feel like I am literally radiating heat from a furnace in my chest. Just taking off a layer of clothes or drinking something cold isn't enough to help. Frigid blowing air is the only thing that makes a dent.

♀ The build up to a hot flash is almost as bad as the hot flash itself. My heart starts to pound. I can feel heat rising in my chest and sweat breaking out on my upper lip and forehead.

♀ During a party at my house on a bitterly cold night, I kept opening a window because I would get so hot. Of course, then everyone else would get cold and ask me to close the window. At one point, after the window had been closed for a while, a friend asked me if I was cold. He thought I was wrapping my arms around my chest to warm myself up. He was rather shocked when I reached into my shirt and pulled out a cold soda can that I had pulled from the fridge and was hugging to my chest! I thought it was a clever alternative to opening up the window again.

♀ Before perimenopause, I couldn't really get my head around the whole hot flash concept. I had hoped I would finally be warm when hot flashes started – and my husband would stop jumping out of bed in reaction to my stone-cold foot snugglies. That's not how it worked out, unfortunately.

♀ What's weird about hot flashes is that there is really no other sensation like them, and you're 40-ish years old or more before you ever experience them. In my pre-peri mindset I thought it might be kind of cool to have one more of life's mysteries left to later years. But reality has set in, and I feel like a gullible teenager all over again. (Yep, the same dopey one who couldn't wait to get her period for the first time.) Now I'm going on 2 years with the thermostat on the fritz and the only life mystery left to look forward to is old age. It's a good thing I keep a lot of chocolate around.

♀ I have had to find a totally different way to dress in order to cover up my sweating from hot flashes. I can't wear silk or anything else that will show dampness. Lightweight, dark colored cotton or knits seem to be the best at both hiding the wet spots and quickly drying. Plus, I keep a jacket or sweater with me to put on after the hot flash is over to camouflage my wet clothes if necessary. I end up feeling cold and clammy sometimes afterwards, but that is better than being embarrassed.

♀ I swear I am going to find a way to strap mini-pads between and under my breasts and on the back of my neck to absorb the sweat during hot flashes!

♀ One day, I had a horrible hot flash. Since I didn't have any tissue or napkins handy to mop up the sweat running down my face, I used a mini-pad that was stashed in my purse. Thank goodness I was in my car and driving down a quiet street so no one could see what I was doing. Now, I make sure I always have tissues with me. I am near the point of getting some handkerchiefs so I have a nice, ladylike way to handle the sweat. If that doesn't work, I might resort to the type of chamois cloth people use to dry their cars. Maybe they make little portable wet vacs?

♀ I just can't drink hot drinks anymore. They almost always trigger a hot flash.

♀ Not only do I sometimes get hot flashes, but I seem to be warmer all the time. I actually enjoy that aspect since I used to be cold most of the time.

♀ Any change in temperature seems to set off my hot flashes.

♀ I can't wear anything but cotton now. If it has even a fraction of wool and I have a hot flash, it feels like sandpaper against my skin. I literally want to rip it off of me.

♀ My girlfriend gave me a pad of sticky notes that say, "Is it hot in here or am I in Hell?" My thoughts, exactly!

♀ How exactly am I supposed to act when I am sitting in a meeting with a group of men and have a hot flash? For years they have listened to me whine about how cold I am all the time. Now I am so hot the sweat is pouring from my forehead. Thankfully they are mostly older guys who must have seen their wives go through this.

♀ Within a few weeks of going on birth control pills to control my symptoms, the hot flashes were almost gone! That was exactly what I was hoping for. Unfortunately, it seems to be short-lived relief. My doctor has had to change my pill three times in the last 18 months to try and keep up with the changes in my hormones.

♀ On the Pill, my periods are back to normal and I don't get hot flashes. I still wake up at night and find that I am hotter than normal, but it doesn't turn into an actual night sweat anymore. I do find that I sweat more than ever before when I exercise, though.

♀ The heat of the hot flash isn't the worst part for me – the anger is. Each time I get a hot flash, I feel so angry that I struggle to control what I say. The heat seems to just melt away my verbal filter.

♀ I've been having hot flashes for several years now. Recently, I've started experiencing intense anxiety before and during the flashes. It feels like a "fight or flight" sensation.

♀ As if a hot flash isn't enough, I get cold chills afterwards. I go from one extreme to the other.

♀ After a hot flash, the back of my neck can be completely soaked. I decided that instead of feeling like I needed to go stick my head under one of those hand drying blowers in the women's room (which would probably trigger yet another hot flash), I would get my hair cut differently so it wouldn't either be wet during a hot flash or limp afterwards. Not only did I solve part of my hot flash related-problems, but I felt like a new "do" really made me feel better about myself! I really like the shorter hair on the sides of my face because it has the added benefit of hiding my crow's feet a little better.

♀ I have started carrying a makeup kit around with me. After a hot flash, I wash or wipe my face, then reapply my makeup. My skin seems better, and I prefer to avoid looking like I've been in a sauna. Yes, I sometimes have to do this multiple times a day and my makeup budget is going up, but I feel better about myself if I look better.

♀ Instead of sticking my head in the freezer, I now go out to my car and blast the air conditioning when I have a particularly bad hot flash. I love the cold air blowing on me! (Just don't do this in a closed garage!)

Crazy Aunt Flo: Strange Periods

We expected irregular periods, but not this early. Of course, you probably thought you would just start to skip periods or go longer in between them. Did you have any idea that you would get wild fluctuations in the amount you bleed, the amount of PMS you experience, and the amount of time you go between periods? Can you believe how different it is every month?

There are as many variations in women's experiences as there are women in the world. Some women report little to no irregularity and a gradual decline in frequency and amount (of course, these are probably the same girls who had perfect skin in high school, who look back in shape 2 weeks after giving birth, or, "can't gain a pound no matter what I eat." Bitches!)

For most women, it is a guessing and worrying game. How long in between, for how many days, how much? These are the times we must arm ourselves with an arsenal of feminine hygiene products at our fingertips at all times. White pants – not so much! Panty liners, mini pads, maxi pads, tampons for light, normal, heavy, super, and gargantuan flow – check! Now we know why women carry such big frickin' purses!

♀ 41, 55, 18. It sounds like a locker combination, but it's not. It's the number of days between my last 3 periods. How the hell do you plan for that except by wearing a pad every single day?

♀ I was so looking forward to the time when I could stop worrying about whether I had a tampon or pad stashed in my purse in case my period started. Now I know I need to have them with me all the time because I never know when I'll need them. If I'm not spotting, I'm gushing. If I'm not bleeding, I'm leaking urine. Actually, I do that when I am bleeding too.

♀ Why didn't anyone tell me that when you stop having regular periods, you still spot at the strangest times, gush unexpectedly, and trickle when you think your period is finally done? I went into this thinking that it would be really nice to start skipping periods and not have to think about it as much. I am shocked to find that I actually think about it more because I never know when it is coming, when it is done, or what will happen in between.

♀ Having false alarms about my period starting is horrible. I'm seriously cramping and discharging, so I repeatedly run to the bathroom to "tampon," but at the moment of truth, nothing red is happening down there. Then, I secretly worry all day that I am dying or something.

♀ I haven't bled through both a tampon and a maxi-pad at the same time since I was a teenager. Now, I have had to throw away pants that got stained.

♀ After going almost 60 days without a period and feeling bloated, sore, hot, and hungry, I took a pregnancy test even though there really didn't seem to be any chance that I could be pregnant unless there had been a massive failure of my very reliable birth control method. I couldn't believe that was the problem, but I was only 41, so I couldn't really think of any alternative. Thank goodness it was negative. It actually took me a while to figure out what was going on. I thought maybe I was stressed or sick. Then I realized. That was my first indication that my hormones were starting to change.

♀ Painful breasts, cramps, and bloating used to signal that my period was coming. Now, my period can come with absolutely no advance warning at all. I can get painful breasts at all different times. And, since I feel bloated most of the time, that's not a signal at all anymore.

♀ I am 46. It has been 9 1/2 months since I have had a period. I don't know whether I should hope my period comes or hope that it doesn't.

♀ Hardly any periods for the last 6 months, then this month, the Hoover Dam has opened. I may bleed to death, but first, I need to run home from work and change my clothes.

♀ I've been wearing a mini-pad every day for months, always expecting that my period will come at some point. I never know what my pre-period symptoms will be these days, so I never know when to expect it. At one point, my nipples were so sore it reminded me of when I was first pregnant. Could I have missed so many periods because I was pregnant? This has never, ever been a PMS symptom but it was my first sign each time I was pregnant. Happily, after a few days of very sore boobs, I got my period. Thank God! Then I realized that I didn't have to wear a pad anymore, at least for a few weeks. Yippee! Oh, nope that won't work. I still have little leakages of pee when I laugh or cough. Damn, I think I am doomed to wear a pad every day for the rest of my life.

♀ I was so surprised at what humongous periods I started to have a few years ago. I thought they would get lighter, not heavier! I can barely cover the bases, so to speak, with super-plus tampons and maxi-pads.

♀ It was the strangest thing. After getting used to my periods coming every few months, I had a period 26 days after my last period, which used to be about normal for me. It was a fairly normal period, too, from a bleeding standpoint. For a few days I wondered why I felt so bloated, kind of crampy, and weird. I didn't figure it out until the last day of my period when I noticed that I felt better. I chuckled over that one! How stupid! I had totally forgotten what a normal period was like.

♀ I am so frigging bloated. I'm tempted to take a needle and pop my belly like a balloon. The bloating used to go away after my period, but now that my periods can be months apart, I spend most of my life feeling like it is about to come.

♀ No one told me that when you stop getting your period on a regular basis, you still feel like you should be getting your period on a regular basis. I still get bloated, crampy, and bitchy, but now it is most of the time instead of just the week or so before my period. I also feel like there is multiple months' worth of blood and tissue saved up in there from missed periods, but when I do finally get a period, hardly anything comes out. I am actually yearning for a real period when everything comes out and my hormones re-adjust. It would be so nice to have that thin, energized, no-worries-about-bleeding feeling that you get a few days after a normal period ends.

♀ It's not enough that they have mini-pads and maxi-pads. They also need to have meno-pads!

♀ My periods have lightened, but it is a really dark, clotty blood. I also feel like there is a different and unpleasant odor. So gross. I can't believe I am actually sharing this info!

♀ I hardly ever get a period any more. When I do get one, it's not the bright red blood that I used to get. It's brown, stringy, and totally disgusting. There have been a couple times when it first comes when I had to wipe both front and back to figure out which end it was coming out of. If this wasn't totally anonymous, I would never tell anyone this!

♀ The color white is gone from anything I wear below the waist. I am totally neurotic about getting my period unexpectedly. I would rather be safe than sorry. Come to think of it, I had better eliminate white on top too. I can't seem to eat a meal these days without getting something on my shirt. What is up with that?

♀ Since I am on the Pill, I get a period every month, but they're getting lighter and lighter. I need to ask my doctor whether I will just stop at the point when I am truly in menopause. I think maybe at that point I have to switch to hormones. I guess I need to talk to my doctor about that, too!

♀ I only get cramps during the "middle" of the month (although, since the time between periods varies so much it is hard to know what is really the middle!). I think it may be when I am ovulating. I even bleed a little. I can just picture my poor tired old ovary trying hard to squeeze out just one more egg. Every time it tries, it is just like *The Little Engine That Could*.

♀ There has to be a payoff for all this crap. Can the periods just end already? Where do I sign up for that?

♀ So I had a few tiny drops of blood in my underwear today. I haven't had a period in over 9 months. Does that count as a period?

♀ For the first few years of perimenopause, everything revolved around when my period was going to come. I was terrified to leave the house, or even to be in the house, without a mini-pad because I never knew when I would start bleeding. My period could come at any time, without any warning, and would just start with a gush. I almost always felt like it could start at any time. Now that I am going several months at a time without a period on a regular basis, I find that I'm not thinking about it so much. I can go weeks without thinking about it, which is a huge relief. I am even willing to go without a pad most of the time. I know that I might get surprised at some point or another, but my periods are so light when they do come now that I doubt I will have a huge accident like I used to have a few years ago. Thank God! I was terrified that I would spend 10 years of my life constantly worrying about getting a period, just like I did during those first few years of puberty!

♀ During the first years of perimenopause, I was constantly upset about the unpredictability in my period. After all those years of expecting it every month, it was so strange not being able to predict it. I worried a lot about getting it unexpectedly. Now that I've been in perimenopause for over five years and hardly ever get a period at all, I can deal with it in a much more relaxed way. When it starts, it starts. I always have a pad in my purse just in case, but I don't worry all the time about when it is going to come. In other words, this is one physical change that gets better over time.

♀ I think that our uteruses (uteri?) and ovaries should just dry up and fall out when they are done being fertile, just like an umbilical cord does. It would certainly make more sense.

Urine Then 'Yer Out: Bladder

Now, here is something so much more fun to discuss, right? If every other commercial on television can be for bladder control products or medication, surely we can talk about it, too. If you are like us, you thought these things were only for really old people, God bless 'em. If so, like us, you'd be wrong (and totally bummed out).

It isn't a problem for everyone, though. If you are one of the lucky ones, we hate you and your dry panties.

♀ My new definition of efficiency: picking up Depends® for my elderly mother, Poise® pads for myself, and Pull-Ups® for my toddler all at the same store and the same time. If this is being in the "sandwich generation," I must be a foot-long hoagie.

♀ I no longer need a watch. I just know that I need to pee every 2 hours, practically on the dot. I feel like a damn egg timer.

♀ I am so proud of my recent great accomplishment: I made it through a whole movie without having to get up to go to pee. Score!

♀ I don't mind that I need to go to the bathroom more frequently. What I do mind is that by the time I realize I need to go to the bathroom, my panties are already damp. It's not even that I get that full. Sometimes after I leak just a little bit, I don't even need to go anymore. Other times, if I can resist the urge for about 15 minutes, the urge goes away. The weird thing is that I never have any problems during the night. I wonder if gravity is part of the problem. I keep seeing those ads for drugs to help urgency and bladder problems, but I don't really want to take medication that has such a long list of side effects that seem worse than the actual problem.

♀ I finally broke down the barrier and got into an executive level position. I am included in big meetings, travel more frequently, and meet frequently with major clients. It's a damn good thing that the old boys club really is that. If I wasn't working with so many older men who tend to have prostate problems and frequently need to take bathroom breaks, I would be in trouble since I can hardly make it more than a couple of hours without having to visit the bathroom. Unfortunately, when I am in a long meeting or with younger clients or business associates, I am like a lunatic trying to find reasons to take breaks. Sometimes I'll even apologize in advance and say that I will need to take a break from a meeting at a certain time for a phone call or arrange for my assistant to call at a certain time to give me updates so I have an excuse to leave the room. The last time I felt like this was when I was pregnant and either had to leave to pee or throw up. Then and now, I'm trying hard to prove myself and my body keeps getting in the way.

♀ I go to the bathroom, feel like I am done, and as soon as I stand up and pull up my pants, squirt! Another few drops involuntarily come out. Argh!

♀ I remember my grandfather being unwilling to go anywhere if he wasn't familiar with the bathroom situation. He had prostate problems. When he needed to go, he needed to go immediately. I feel the same exact way now. I am constantly scoping out where the restrooms are and scheduling my day to make sure I'm near one on a regular basis. It seems to be taking up a lot more of my time than it should.

♀ Even the way I pee has changed. It used to come out in a strong, steady stream. Now it sort of trickles out. It doesn't go straight into the toilet either. It dribbles down over my perineum. I think that just contributes to the overall dryness and discomfort of that region.

♀ I used to love the summer baseball season, watching my boy play. Now, I pray to whatever deity will listen that I won't have to pee during the game. They only have the port-o-potties. Everything is working against me in there. I am short, I don't want my purse, clothes, or body to touch the floor, the seat, or the sides, I am trying not to breathe, and my pee, for some strange reason, now likes to squirt sideways making it almost impossible to predict the landing point!

♀ It seems like I have to pee more when I drink caffeinated coffee in the morning. I figured it out because in the afternoon I can go much longer without having to go to the bathroom, even if I have been drinking water or soda. In the morning, even if I don't drink much coffee, I still have to go repeatedly. When I stick to decaf, I seem to do much better.

♀ I have resorted to drinking less so I have to pee less. It seems to be helping a little bit.

♀ My girlfriend told me she read that some problems with urine leaking have to do with weak pelvic floor muscles. I was willing to try anything to help, so I started going to Pilates and really focusing on my core strength and pelvic floor. Not only did my urinary problems get a bit better, but I feel like my stomach has gotten a bit flatter, too. A two-fer! I have a feeling if I keep going, I will start to see some other improvements, too. I don't love exercising, but I do love the results, whether you can see them or not!

♀ Using vaginal hormone cream, which my doctor prescribed to combat vaginal dryness, has actually helped my urinary control issues. I can now make it to the bathroom in time ... most of the time.

Waisted Space: Stomach/Waist

There are some key aspects of perimenopause that are similar to pregnancy: you never know how you will feel next and your body seems like it is constantly changing, especially in the mid-section.

♀ I had gotten used to that "pooch" on my lower stomach, that area of extra skin that looks like hail damage that was a left-over of pregnancy. But all of a sudden I have put on a ton of weight around my middle. Is this what they mean by a "spare tire?" I actually think it is more like a life preserver. I have never gained weight in those areas before. My whole body shape is changing.

♀ I used to have a great waistline. Now I won't even tuck in a shirt. I now understand why all the clothes at stores that target middle-aged women have poufy, loose shirts, and jackets. It's not that middle-aged women suddenly *want* clothes like that – they *need* clothes like that!

♀ My gut is expanding! Ugh! This is so painful to me. Despite my workouts, controlling the carbs, and watching my overall calories, it seems like I am about to give birth to triplets! Strange, they've been gestating for about 2 years now.

♀ The other day as I was getting out of the shower, my husband looked at me and said, "Your ass moved around to the front." His funeral was lovely.

♀ My trainer looked at me with sympathetic eyes and told me, "Menopause just makes women thicker around the middle." It was so matter of fact. So final. So blunt. I guess it is better that I should just go out and buy bras that are size 36 instead of 34 and pants that are a size bigger, but it would be nice to have at least a little hope, especially from the person I pay to help me stay in shape, that things could get better if I work at it. I would think she would want to give me some hope so I keep coming and working out with her.

♀ It seems the combination of birth control pills to control my moods and strange periods, Zoloft® to control my depression, and overall stress have combined to produce the amount of weight I gained when I was 9 months pregnant. I can't go off the medications, and I don't see the stress going away. I am just going to try really hard not to worry about the weight right now.

♀ Going shopping is incredibly frustrating because I just can't figure out what will look good on me now. If I go with the old stand-bys, the stuff that has always looked good on me in the past, I get home and realize how horrible I look.

27

♀ Am I just supposed to give in and get used to this strange new shape I have? How long does it take to adjust to having a different "me" looking back in the mirror, to knowing that people see an older woman, to not having guys' heads turn my way, to having to buy entirely different types of clothes? For me, how my body looks, not the physical symptoms, is the hardest part of this transition.

♀ I am starting to wish I lived in the times when women wore corsets to cinch in their waists! If all that extra flesh could be squeezed up into the bust, I would be in great shape. Oh, or how about the times when curvy, voluptuous women were considered the most beautiful?

♀ I am in shape! Oval is a shape, right?

♀ Now that I understand how a woman's shape changes during the time before menopause, I feel like I can look at a woman and have a pretty good idea of whether or not she is in perimenopause.

♀ I was having lunch the other day with two male co-workers when a woman walked by and they both said "muffin top" and snickered. When I asked what a muffin top was, they explained that it's a commonly used term for a girl when she has fat hanging over the waistline of her pants – like the top of a muffin. Now I find myself paranoid that I might have a muffin top! (The ironic part is how they are both sitting back in the booth with these big bellies talking about how the women look. Oh, it must be good to be a man.)

♀ About 10 years ago, my sister-in-law, who is about 15 years older, went clothes shopping with me. I will never forget how horrified I was when she told me, as I modeled something fairly tight, that I should enjoy being able to wear those types of tight clothes while I could because as you get older, you get bulgy on your back at the bra line and can't do anything about it. She was in great shape and didn't have any bulges anywhere else, so I figured she knew what she was talking about. I put it out of my mind, though, because those days seemed far in the future for me. Now, when I put on a shirt that is somewhat tight and check in the mirror to see if my back bulges are showing, I think of her. I guess I am glad she warned me so that I would know to check. When I see women with skin bulging out around their bra straps, I figure they probably don't even realize it because they don't think to check for it.

♀ I haven't gained a pound and my exercise routine is the same, but my mid-section is just tons flabbier. I feel like I am overflowing the top of my jeans.

♀ I am gaining weight even though I am not eating any more or exercising any less.

♀ My strategy has been to eat anything and everything I want, and then make it up with exercise. Eating good food reduces stress, exercise reduces stress and keeps me fit – personally, I think it is genius!

♀ I have never been a big eater, but I have suddenly become hungrier than I have ever been in my life. Not only am I craving food, which I don't normally do, but I am craving foods that I don't normally eat.

♀ I love the line in *Menopause The Musical*® about how the woman's appetite hasn't changed at all – during the day. I have the worst night-time food cravings. Actually, they aren't food cravings. I get food desperation. I will shovel anything I can get my hands on into my mouth.

♀ I always craved chocolate around my period. Now I crave it all the time. I think that maybe instead of hormones I should take chocolate in pill form.

To Sleep, Perchance to Dream: Sleep

As if losing your ability to function well during the day wasn't enough (you'll read more about this in Section IV), you might also find that you don't do as well during the night, either. Sleep disturbances are common during this time of life. Be prepared not just to wake up in a hot sweat but also to wake up just for no reason at all. Like so many other aspects of perimenopause, there is just no way to tell how you'll be affected or how long it will last. We do know, though, that when you have trouble sleeping through the night, it makes it much harder to cope with everything else.

♀ I used to be a great sleeper. It was my way of decompressing and coping with difficulties in my life. Now, lack of sleep is one of my biggest difficulties. I just can't get through the night and sometimes I can't even fall asleep at all. If I'm not waking up soaked with sweat, I am running to the bathroom. Sometimes I just wake up and can't get back to sleep.

♀ I feel like a new mother, only instead of waking up to change the baby, I am waking up to change myself out of drenched nightgowns. When I was a new mom, I learned to go back to sleep pretty quickly. Now I lie awake and can't get back to sleep.

♀ I'm sleeping fine, but for the first time since I was pregnant, I'm having incredibly vivid, dynamic, and complicated dreams. Even though I have slept, I still feel tired when I wake up in the morning.

♀ I sleep all night long, but I don't feel rested at all.

♀ My worries about sleep are only making things worse. I am so tense about sleeping, I think it is actually contributing to my sleep problems. I am in a vicious cycle.

♀ I am learning that I just have different biorhythms these days. I get a sudden burst of energy at about 11 at night. Sometimes when I wake up early in the morning and can't fall back to sleep, I do better if I get out of bed and get things done. Then, if I am sleepy after I get home from work in the afternoon or on a weekend, I try to take a nap. I'll take sleep whenever I can get it.

♀ I think a lot of my moodiness is related to being tired and stressed about being tired. I also think my daytime forgetfulness could be related to my exhaustion.

♀ My doctor prescribed sleeping pills. I resisted taking them unless I hadn't slept well in 2 weeks, and even then I felt guilty and worried about taking them. The next time I went in for an appointment, I admitted that I still wasn't sleeping well. She told me to take them every night for a while to get back in the habit of sleeping. I have been doing it for a few weeks and feel tons better. I don't want to stay on them for much longer, but I am glad I have done it for a while. I'm going to wean myself off them and hope that I can sleep without them. Well, maybe tomorrow I will... Or next week ...

♀ I was absolutely desperate for a good night's sleep, but since I am the only adult in the house, I was afraid to take a sleeping pill. One night, I had just had enough and couldn't take it anymore and decided to take a sleeping pill. I told my kids that if they needed me, they would have to come into my room and get me. If the house was on fire, they would need to call 911.

♀ I was really relieved to read online that problems with sleep are the most bothersome and frequent symptoms of the time before menopause. I don't like it, but at least I know I am not imagining things.

♀ When I just can't turn my brain off enough to relax and get to sleep, I play Internet games. My favorite is timed, has addictive sound effects, and gives me this strange sense of accomplishment when I get to higher levels. Best of all, it stops my brain from racing while I am playing. While I sometimes find myself at my computer until the wee hours of the night (or morning), it relaxes me to the point that I can finish a game, dash to bed, and keep my brain empty long enough to fall asleep for at least a little while.

What to Try: To Adjust to Typical Physical Changes

✓ If irregular periods are really bothering you, talk to your doctor. Birth control pills might be an option to regulate your cycle.

✓ Carry a hair tie or clip in your purse to put up your hair during or after a hot flash. It may not look good, but it will keep you from cutting off the back of your hair with the closest pair of scissors because you can't stand the feel of it on your neck during the "boil."

✓ Switch to waterproof or long-lasting makeup so it doesn't all run down your face during a hot flash.

✓ Wear cotton and other breathable fabrics whenever possible.

✓ Increase the amount of soy in your diet since it is said to decrease hot flashes. Soy milk and edamame are good additions if you aren't in love with tofu. Maybe it will help and maybe it won't, but unless you are allergic, it might be worth a try!

✓ Try reducing the amount of caffeine in your diet to see if it reduces the number or severity of hot flashes. This might help you sleep better, too.

✓ Track the triggers that set off your hot flashes. Alcohol, wool clothes, hot drinks, and other external factors may play a role. Once you know your personal triggers, you can try to avoid them and cut down on the number of hot flashes you experience.

✓ Keep a small battery-powered fan in your purse.

✓ Sleep on a towel and keep extra pajamas next to your bed. If you wake up drenched, it will be faster and easier to change, get dry, and fall back to sleep faster.

✓ If you are experiencing urinary incontinence, talk to your doctor about whether prescription medication might help.

✓ If you are leaking urine, use incontinence pads rather than panty-liners for periods. They will absorb better and minimize odor. If you are embarrassed to buy them, go to a store that has a self-checkout or order them online for delivery to your door. Or, tell the check-out guy that they are for your elderly grandmother! Or, make your husband do it. It's the least he can do, right?

✓ Maintaining the strength of your pelvic floor can help with stress incontinence. Kegel exercises, where you squeeze your pelvic floor like you do to stop urine flow, can help. Do them when you're in the car at a stoplight, in the shower, doing your other exercises, whatever.

✓ Your body is changing, so maybe your exercise routine needs to change too. What worked before might not be right now. Perhaps adjusting the amount of cardio and/or weight training will help.

✓ Your new body shape may not change. Wear clothes that make the most of it so you are comfortable and good about yourself. Get rid of the clothes that make you feel bad.

✓ Try to find something to do right before bedtime that calms you enough to relax. Maybe it is doing a crossword puzzle, reading, knitting, watching TV shows that don't make you think, or taking a bath. Maybe it is good sex ... then again, probably not. It might be time to change your routine a bit to find something that works for you now.

✓ Consider taking sleep aids. Prescription sleeping pills, "PM" versions of over-the-counter pain medicine, or natural products, such as valerian or melatonin, might work. If the first thing you try doesn't work, try something else. Remember to check with your doctor for suggestions and guidance.

Chapter 3

You Aren't Imagining It – *Surprising* Physical Changes

Dear Mother Nature: People have this idea of you as this peaceful, maternal creature creating beauty on Earth. Well I am seeing a whole other side of you. I think you might want to consider a few years on the shrink's chair to help you figure out why you like to torture women.

I knew there would be at least a few unexpected aspects of the "change," but, you just keep surprising me — throwing something new into the mix, reminding me who's really in charge.

You've read books, talked with your mother or other female relatives, seen *Menopause The Musical*®, and/or observed the generations before you. You might have expected the mood swings, hot flashes, sleep disturbances, and continence issues, not to mention the irregular periods. You may not even be surprised to see some wrinkles, need reading glasses, or need to stock up on KY™. Unfortunately, Mother Nature still has some real surprises up her sleeve.

It is important to recognize that some of the physical changes described in this chapter can't necessarily be attributed to hormonal changes. Some can just be related to good, old-fashioned aging. It's irrelevant to us whether something like having skin that has the texture of crepe paper is directly related to perimenopause or is just a sign of the times during which perimenopause occurs. We just want to get as many of the possible changes out there in the open so you won't be blind-sided by them, think you are imagining things, or feel alone and frustrated.

Facing the Music: Face

We all expect to look older over the years. Many of us probably expect that the first real signs of aging will show on our faces during this time in our lives, so that is no surprise. You might be surprised, however, at how the changes seem to happen so fast and that there's so much more than just a few wrinkles here and there.

♀ I have a new fascination with all the plastic surgery shows on TV. I was never interested before and really thought that those women were being totally silly. Now that I can see a clear difference when I pull back the skin on my face, I am starting to understand. If I feel like if I already need help in my mid-40's, how am I going to look in my 50's and 60's? My face is going to be as saggy as my boobs! Maybe I should start my surgery savings fund now.

♀ I have a strategy for looking better. I grew my hair out and pull it back tightly into a ponytail. The tension on my hair gives my skin some support and acts like a mini-face-lift! Unless I start losing my hair, like some of my friends have, I'm set!

♀ So exactly which crease on my eyelid is the one where I am supposed to apply the eye shadow that is labeled for the crease? The place I used to consider the crease is now part of my lower lid, and there is skin hanging over where the crease used to be. And, when I do brush on the eye shadow, it takes awhile for the skin to go back to its usual place on my eyelid.

♀ I feel like my mother is stalking me. I see her when I am strolling through the mall, when I turn the corner in my bathroom, and when I get my hair cut. Every time I look in a mirror the face that looks back seems like it should be my mother, not me.

♀ It is clearly time to get out the spackle. My old makeup just can't cope with the dark tints around my eyes and upper lip. My first step was to buy concealer, which I will continue to use, but it isn't enough. I now need true, heavy foundation. I used to think that kind of makeup looked like a mask. Now, I feel like my natural skin looks like a mask, so I need to hide it.

♀ I am seeing a stranger and stranger image looking back at me in the mirror every day. I wonder what other people are seeing when they look at me.

♀ My medicine cabinet is no longer big enough. I have a lovely new basket of lotions and potions designed for smoothing wrinkles, brightening the skin around the eyes, reducing puffiness, and creating a more even skin tone. My routine each morning and evening has gotten much longer!

♀ Not only have I needed new skin care products, but I have also had to change my makeup. I have found that using lighter, matte products, rather than heavier or shimmery products, helps take the focus off the little lines and wrinkles that have crept up on me.

♀ Suddenly, I have zits just like I did as a teenager – big, cyst-like bumps that take forever to go away. I love sharing most things with my teenagers, but sharing pimple cream isn't one of them!

♀ I have always had to deal with acne. After a prolonged period without my period, my face was completely clear. It was awesome. Then, when my period came, I broke out again. If getting rid of hormones means getting rid of my pimples, I will be thrilled!

♀ My face seems to be holding up fairly well, but I am getting a chicken neck. I see a lot of turtleneck sweaters in my future.

♀ While everything else on my body seems to be getting thicker, my lips are getting thinner. The tiny wrinkles all around my mouth just seem to be pointing to them, too. I have invested in thicker lip lining pencils, lip plumping lipsticks, and anything else I can find to help the problem. If I ever decide to have cosmetic surgery on my lips, it's fortunate that there will be plenty of fat from elsewhere on my body to plump them up!

♀ A group of girlfriends and I were sitting together at the table at a Bar Mitzvah party for the son of another friend. We were talking about how time flies and how amazed we were to be at this stage of life. We started talking about whether we had cried at the event since this was the last kid in our group to hit this milestone. I said that everyone probably thought I had, but I really just had a runny nose that wouldn't stop. I couldn't believe the reaction. Every woman there started talking about how runny her nose has been lately. Each said that at first she thought she had a cold or allergies, then over time realized that her nose was just permanently runny. It seems we now know why older women always used to carry tissues tucked in their sleeves!

♀ I have dental floss and toothpicks in my car, my purse, and my desk at work. I can't believe how much food gets stuck in my teeth these days. Maybe it is because my gums are receding? I can tell they are because there are several places with a new-found sensitivity to temperature and touch. I can also see the difference.

♀ I was going crazy trying to figure out why I had a dry, bitter taste in my mouth. I switched mouthwash and toothpaste, which seemed to help, but only a little bit. I starting keeping a drink with me at all times. Then, I mentioned something to my girlfriend about it. Apparently, she has been dealing with the same thing. Chalk it up to perimenopause, I guess.

♀ You know how older people tend to spit when they talk? Well recently my girlfriends and I have noticed that we are doing it more now, too. I just can't imagine what is happening with our lips that could make this happen. Is it that we are producing more saliva? How unfair would that be considering how dry all of the other places that are supposed to be moist are!

Don't Judge a Book by its Cover: Skin

Think about how often you hear about women who say they go on hormones to keep their skin looking young. Did you think they were doing that just to avoid wrinkles? We did! Now, you will find out the truth. Loss of hormones can make the skin all over your body become loose, dry, itchy, scaly, thin, and blotchy in addition to wrinkly. Ugh.

♀ About half of my wardrobe is off limits. Either it is too uncomfortable on my itchy skin, will show off how dry my skin is, or will show rolls of loose skin. The rest of my wardrobe doesn't fit. I may just have to wear pajamas and sweatpants the rest of my life.

♀ The texture of my skin seems to be getting worse by the minute. I am trying new creams, scrubs, and makeup to try to hide it or fix it. I wonder if I could get a full-body chemical peel.

♀ One of the most irritating new symptoms is just feeling creepy, crawly all over. It's not exactly an itch, but that is the closest word I can use.

♀ When I take my clothes off, lots of little flakes of dead skin come off, too. It is absolutely disgusting. I am going through twice the amount of lotion I used to, but am still dry and itchy. I know I live in a dry climate, but this is ridiculous. It is much worse than it has ever been before.

♀ I have lotion stashed in my car, on my desk, in my bathroom, in my closet, and by the kitchen sink. Sometimes my hands are so dry they hurt. I also get scratched so easily because my skin is so dry.

♀ My skin feels like it's a size too big. It is sagging and loose all over my body, even in weird places like in my armpits and between my breasts. I hate seeing myself in the mirror when I get in or out of the shower. It frustrates me that no matter what I weigh or how toned my muscles are, my skin still doesn't feel tight.

♀ One of my secret pleasures is watching a reality show about brides choosing their wedding dresses. On the last episode, a girl tried on a dress that was too big, so they used big clips all down the back of the dress to pull it in tight. I want that done on my skin all up and down my back, from my head to my ankles!

♀ I can't stand that my skin is getting covered in little tiny wrinkles. It's not just on my face either. I notice it in the crook of my elbow, on my neck, and between my breasts.

♀ I feel like someone covered me in wrapping paper for the wrong holiday. I look in the mirror and feel like I have aged 10 years in 10 months. I wish I could just rip off my skin and find something wonderful underneath.

♀ The crepe-like skin and droopiness of my eyelids is actually better after using a product that is specifically for improving the firmness and brightness of eyelids. The dark, puffy area under my eyes is even better. I can't believe it. You can't compare it to plastic surgery, but this is good enough for me.

♀ I like to think that I am working on improving my posture and grace. Really what I am doing is trying to hold my head and chin(s) high to hide the saggy skin on my jaw and neck!

Beauty Is in the Eye of the Beholder: Eyes

Changes in our eyesight are something we expect as we get older. It might be just aging, or it might be that hormones affect the eyes as much as they affect everything else. Dry eyes are a common complaint for "women our age" according to our eye doctor. As if we need one more thing to dry up? As usual, we don't care what causes the changes. We just want to confirm that it's really happening!

♀ I never used to understand why people used magnifying makeup mirrors. Now I get it. You start to get whiskers at exactly the same time you stop being able to see them in a regular mirror.

♀ I rationalized that I was going to the high-end grocery store to look for really good vitamins for my inability to focus on words, my sudden lack of brainpower, and my hot flashes. Of course, while I was there, I knew I would "see" the display in the same aisle as the menopause supplements – the little reader glasses. After doing my best to read the bottles of supplements to see which could help, I realized that the ability to see clearly might have a positive effect on my ability to process the information provided in what had suddenly become fuzzy little letters. After slinking over to the display and trying on a few pairs with different levels of magnification, I realized that they really did help. I could see and read what was on the bottles. I left the store with new glasses, 3 bottles of vitamins and minerals, and a book about hormones.

♀ Reading has always been my greatest pleasure. My book group meetings were sacred on the family schedule. Suddenly, reading wasn't pleasurable anymore. For about a year, I kept complaining that I just couldn't find books that could keep my attention. Had I read all the good books already? Had publishers suddenly lost track of what readers wanted? Had my interests changed that much? When it became harder and harder to read menus, pill bottles, and instructions on the side of packaged foods, I decided that the time had finally come for me to get reading glasses. They helped so much that I decided to try them when I was reading, not just looking at a box or bottle. Lo and behold, reading suddenly got much easier and more interesting when I could actually see the words more clearly. I wish I had figured this out months ago. I am back to reading like normal. With everything else that is changing in my body and my world right now, I am relieved to have this simple pleasure back, even if I can't do it unless I have my glasses with me. I absolutely refuse, however, to ever put them on a chain around my neck. I would rather have pairs stashed all over my house and office, no matter how often I forget where I put them.

♀ The movie *Sex and the City* made me feel so good. Even Charlotte and Carrie were having trouble seeing. Charlotte, of course, had adorable glasses. Carrie just uses Big's or holds things far away to see.

♀ I love my electronic book reader. On a good day, I can have the font on one of the smaller sizes. On a normal day, I have it set on a medium size. On a bad day, late in the evening when my eyes are tired, or when my reading glasses (all 12 pairs) are lost, I put it on the large size. They should highlight that feature when they are marketing them and millions of women my age would buy them!

♀ I thought I was aging really gracefully. I even took it well when I realized that I needed to get progressive lenses (a kinder word for bifocals or trifocals) so I could see near and far. The new glasses are great. But, I what I hadn't seen before were the wrinkles forming at the edges of my eyes, the sandpaper-like skin on my hands and arms, or the grey hairs sprouting in some really unfortunate places. Maybe I will go back to my old glasses....

♀ Although most of the time my eyes feel drier and scratchier than they used to, I occasionally just start tearing up in one eye. It is really strange because the tears just keep coming but, instead of feeling like just tears, my eye feels sort of sticky. It happens at the weirdest times for no apparent reason.

♀ My girlfriends and I were having a great time discussing the bizarre experiences we've been having. We were discussing all the usual suspects, such as weight gain, crazy periods, and vaginal dryness, when eye problems came up. We weren't even that surprised to find that all of us had experienced not just changes in vision, but also dry eyes. I was totally shocked, though, when I mentioned that I thought my eyes seemed drier when I use eye-liner, even though I have used eye-liner on and off since I was 13. You should have heard the shrieks of agreement. All of them said they thought the same thing, but hadn't really felt like it was something tangible enough to consider a symptom of perimenopause. However, if everyone in a group of women who are all experiencing hormone changes is experiencing the same strange thing, I think it counts.

♀ I was just reading an article about eye changes in the newsletter of one of the largest and most respected national menopause societies. It talked about how dry eyes and blurred vision are common symptoms of menopause and goes on to discuss other eye-related changes that women in their 50's and 60's are likely to experience. First of all, are they discussing "true" menopause, after periods stop, or could it also apply to perimenopause? I wish these articles would be clear. I just recently started perimenopause, but my eyes are driving me crazy. Is it related or not? Should I be reading articles about menopause or just about perimenopause?

♀ When the lighting is even the least little bit dim, I have the hardest time focusing. It makes it very difficult in restaurants, in particular, when I have trouble reading the menu.

♀ I've always felt bad for older women who have their makeup on like they are circus clowns with big, round, red circles on their cheeks, lipstick out of bounds, and mascara all over their eyelids. I figured they had just lost the energy to be careful about how they applied their makeup or were trying to cover their wrinkles by using a lot of it. But, after putting my makeup on at a hotel that had better light than my own bathroom, I realized that I might have been looking a lot like them when I put on my makeup at home. I obviously couldn't see what I was doing. As soon as I got home from vacation, I went out and bought a light up mirror with magnification.

♀ I can't believe that I am sitting around talking with my girlfriends about the relative benefits of bifocals versus progressive lenses versus reading glasses. It makes me feel so old.

♀ How can I possibly go to the eye doctor and get glasses? It seems like my vision changes from day to day.

♀ My eye doctor just told me that it is normal for people my age to have trouble shifting from focusing on something far away to something close. I was really relieved because I couldn't figure out how he was going to prescribe glasses when I can see near and far, but it takes me time to adjust from one to the other. Of course, I wish there was something he could do to help other than just reassure me by telling me that at sometime in the future I will need bifocals.

Bosom Buddies: Breasts

Sure, you knew the girls might start getting a bit droopy at our age, but that is only the start! Some other common changes may be a bit more surprising. Remember, we warned you!

Important note: While it is easy and somewhat comforting to attribute every change in your body to perimenopause, it is not always the cause. If you have a symptom that is making you nervous or is only in one breast, check with your doctor. Also make sure you know the symptoms of breast cancer, stay on track with your scheduled mammograms, and perform regular self-examinations. While you can get breast cancer at virtually any age, this is the time to be extra diligent about your breast health.

♀ My breasts used to be the harbinger of my period. A few days before my period started, my breasts would get achy and sore. Now, I can have periods without having any breast tenderness, or I can have breast tenderness without any periods. I liked having my signal system and am frustrated that I can't count on it anymore. I also don't like having my breasts ache for days on end with no outcome! At least when I knew my period was coming, there was a point.

♀ Breast tenderness was always my signal that my period was about to come. Now, after a double mastectomy, I don't have that signal anymore. Combine that with perimenopause, when my periods are all over the place. I have absolutely no idea at all when I will get a period.

♀ My breasts and nipples have been tender for over a month. The last time I felt like this was when I was first pregnant and felt like my breasts were already a size bigger. They definitely aren't bigger now, but they feel like they are swollen.

♀ Not only are my boobs sore on a fairly regular basis, but I actually have the sensation of "let-down" like when I was nursing my babies. Never in a million years did I expect to have that feeling ever again. I didn't like it then, and I don't like it now.

♀ My nipples are so dry and itchy. I took off a black camisole yesterday and had two circles of boob dandruff on the inside! I wonder if they make "Boob and Shoulders" shampoo? Although, I guess it would be more like Boob and Belly. How much more humiliating can this get?

♀ Hairy, saggy, itchy boobs. Lovely. Just lovely. I had absolutely no idea they could change this much this fast.

♀ I have decided to turn putting lotion on my very dry breasts into a form of foreplay. It is so much more fun when my husband does it! If it morphs into putting lotion onto other parts of my body or lubricant where needed, so be it!

♀ My nipples seem a lot less sensitive sexually these days. When my husband touches them, it just doesn't do anything for me anymore.

♀ Not only do I not get turned on when my husband tries to touch my breasts, but it is actually sort of irritating.

♀ I'm not sure whether it is because I have gained a little bit of weight, but my breasts seem to be bigger. Unfortunately, that just means that they are saggier, too.

♀ I was watching *The View* the other day and heard Whoopi Goldberg refer to her boobs as "Snoopy noses." It still makes me laugh every time I think about it.

♀ I have itty, bitty titties, but I am still getting stretch marks on them because they are getting so saggy. First of all, I didn't know you could even get stretch marks there unless you are well-endowed or overweight; secondly, I thought I would get to avoid droopy boobs since mine are so small. No such luck, apparently.

♀ My breasts aren't just drooping, they are also moving to the side. Although the fibroid cysts in my breasts sometimes hurt (especially if I have more than just a little bit of caffeine), I think they are about the only thing giving me any fullness at all! If they go away after I am through menopause, I hate to think how soft and saggy I will be!

♀ Cleavage is a thing of the past. When I lie down on my back, my boobs are in my armpits. Yuck.

♀ My breasts seem to have moved around to my back. I now have pads of fat on my back under the band of my bra.

♀ I had a great boob job about 15 years ago. My breasts are just as perky now as they were back then. Unfortunately, the skin around then and between them is getting wrinkly and saggy. I look great if I keep covered up, but I worry that I look really strange in a tank top or bathing suit.

♀ I went bra shopping the other day because my reliable old bras just weren't cutting it any more. I was literally in tears in the dressing room. Every time I put on a bra, there was saggy, baggy skin hanging over the edges under my arms and just in front of my armpits. No more pretty little lacy things for me, apparently. I needed to leave the cute bra store and hit the functional bra section of a department store. I ended up with ugly, full coverage bras that extend all the way out to my arms instead of just being on my breasts.

♀ My bras don't fit like they used to. I am down to one comfy bra that I wear all the time. I know I need to go buy new ones but don't really want to go through that agony.

♀ I finally decided that I can no longer shop for bras at stores that cater to supermodels. I went to a store where they helped me find a bra that properly fits around my torso and gives the right amount of support, not to mention the right cup size. When I chose a bra that was the right size and had some padding, I felt like the girls were finally standing up at attention.

♀ I have decided to be like Carrie Bradshaw in *Sex and the City*. I will never take my bra off in front of a man again! Me in a pretty bra is much more attractive than me with saggy breasts.

♀ I found a lifting and firming potion that actually seems to be working on my face. My mother thought I had gotten my eyebrows waxed, but it was really just that the skin on my eyelids wasn't sagging so much. I think I'll buy the stuff in bulk and spread it on my boobs to see if it works there, too! If it does, my butt is next.

♀ I am thinking about giving up bras all together. They are itchy, pinchy, pokey, and the straps are too loose or too tight. Besides the fact that they are too frickin' hot and I collect so much sweat underneath my boobs that I am thinking there might be some sort of a leak somewhere!

The Vagina Dialogues: Vagina

Our vaginas: that hidden, oh-so-private, not to be discussed part of our bodies. Sure, we talk about our sex lives and our periods, but, unless we are recovering from delivering a baby or suffering from a yeast infection, we rarely talk about our actual vaginas. Well, it's time to break that taboo. Say "vagina" (not "va-jay-jay" or "hoo-ha") three times out-loud and get used to it. Louder!

How about vulva? Did you know that we often use the term vagina when we are actually referring to the vulva? Let's clear it up right here and now. A woman's vulva is actually all of the external sexual organs of the crotch including the opening to the vagina, the clitoris, the labia (majora and minora), the urethra, and the area over the pelvic bone. The vagina is the internal structure that connects the vulva to the uterus. You can see that the two are most often used incorrectly. Who knew?

The vagina/vulva are amazing body parts that, when all is going well, you can pretty much ignore. But when hormones start changing during perimenopause, you just may not be able to ignore that area any longer. Suddenly, it may seem like a separate part of your body that just isn't in sync with everything else. It starts demanding attention – and not necessarily the good kind!

♀ I apologized to my husband for my body's recent inability to respond even when I am in the mood. I told him that I feel like I don't even know my vagina anymore. His response was that he is very familiar with it and happy to tell me anything I need to know. This is very sweet, of course, but not exactly helpful. How can such an intimate part of me feel so totally disconnected and unpredictable? It is so frustrating when it doesn't respond when it should.

♀ Lately, I've been feeling like my cervix is hanging down into my vagina. Turns out, it is! My doctor says uterine prolapse is not uncommon for "women my age" (God, I hate that phrase!) as everything inside tends to sag (along with everything on the outside). The good news is that my uterine fibroids are so big that they are preventing any further sagging. I guess that is good news...

♀ I totally expected vaginal dryness at this age. I figured that is why there are so many ads on TV these days for lubricants. Little did I know that vaginal dryness is something that can make you uncomfortable all the time, not just during sex. No wonder this is something that even my mother couldn't keep quiet about.

♀ Being so dry is drastically affecting my sex life. The idea of sex just sounds painful, not fun.

♀ I mentioned to my doctor that I was experiencing bad vaginal dryness. He said that it is normal and proceeded to discuss "vaginal atrophy." I was so shocked that I didn't pay attention. So, when I got home, I looked it up on the Internet to see what I missed. Up popped a very close up picture of an old woman's vagina with the doctor's fingers holding the labia open to show the narrowed vaginal opening. Good God! It turns out we can expect to be dry, have the skin in our vagina thin out, and have the opening narrow. That scares me to death, not to mention grosses me out. By the way, apparently we can go somewhat bald and gray down there as we get older, too!

♀ I was aware that it was possible to dry up and close up inside. I am shocked and dismayed to find that you can get saggy and loose on the outside at the same time. Seems sort of unfair, don't you think?

♀ My doctor literally told me that as women get older, they have to "use it or lose it." The doctor suggests regular sex to avoid vaginal atrophy and promote better vaginal lubrication. My husband would be happy to hear that, although I won't tell him! Having sex is the very last thing I want right now. I sometimes even bleed afterwards!

♀ I sort of expected to get dry inside and have to use lubricant for sex. I had no idea how dry I could be all the time, though. My perineum is so dry it gets cracked and bleeds. When I pee, I have to pat myself dry rather than wipe because wiping is so uncomfortable. I am also incredibly itchy inside. I checked with my doctor, who said it is just dryness, not an infection. Good news, but at least with an infection you can take medicine to make things better.

♀ When I was cleaning out my grandmother's apartment after she passed away, I found a stash of vaginal Premarin® cream. Could it really be possible for vaginal dryness or atrophy to remain a problem until you are in your 90's? No wonder old ladies can be so cranky.

♀ I have had more vaginal infections in the last few years than I have had in all the previous years put together. My doctor says it is because the hormone changes cause changes in the acidity level in my vagina. At least there is a reason.

♀ For 2 months I walked around feeling like I could literally scratch my vagina out if I wasn't careful. I was so intensely dry and itchy. I had absolutely no discharge, no odor, no nothing other than intense itching and dryness so bad that I was cracking and bleeding inside and out. Since I didn't have any other symptoms, I figured it wasn't an infection. I tried all sorts of over-the-counter vaginal creams and lotions. Some helped a little. Even my butt was getting itchy, so I added hemorrhoid cream to the mix. It would get better for a few days; then it would get worse again. Finally, I decided to try medicine for yeast infection, just in case, before calling the doctor and going in for an appointment. I could totally feel the medicine working as soon as I put it in. Don't make my mistake of attributing everything to perimenopausal symptoms. Sure, that was probably the reason why I got a yeast infection for the first time in over 25 years, but that alone wasn't the cause of my discomfort. I didn't need to suffer for so long.

♀ I hate being so aware of my vagina for so much of the time. If it was because I was feeling sexy and in the mood, that would be one thing, but it's not. I am just so uncomfortable down there. It almost feels like the skin inside my vagina is burned, and nothing seems to help.

♀ I don't have a vaginal infection, but I sometimes feel a kind of stinging, itchy pain deep inside.

♀ Lately, just when my period is starting, I get a prickly feeling deep inside. While I have learned to use this uncomfortable feeling as a sign that my period is starting, since all the other signs that I used to count on no longer occur, it actually hurts sometimes.

♀ I have found that my vaginal dryness feels better after having sex. Maybe the extra blood flow to that region helps. Maybe semen is a natural lubricant. I don't know and don't care. As long as I use lube, this is a good reason to have sex even if I am not really in the mood. Sex as therapy isn't exactly my idea of a good time, but my husband hasn't seemed to notice or care!

♀ I have tried vaginal hormone cream, oral estrogen, and homeopathic treatments for the vaginal dryness that I started to experience once my periods got to the point when they were almost non-existent. This is not just about sex. I am so uncomfortable I can barely sit down for more than a few minutes. When I walk I feel like I have sandpaper inside me. I think I need to switch my doctor, not just treatments. The one I have now just doesn't seem to take this seriously enough.

♀ Putting tampons in for a few days every month was bad enough. Lately I have been using an anti-itch cream almost every day, sometimes multiple times a day. I recently added vaginal moisturizer, which is better because it has an applicator so I don't have to put it on by hand. Now I have a prescription for estrogen cream that has to be put on every day for 2 weeks, then once or twice a week. I thought I was going to be able to pay less attention to my vagina, not more, as my periods decreased.

♀ Thank goodness for vaginal hormone cream. It made me feel like myself again down there. I don't love putting it in, but the results are worth it.

♀ I never thought I would be happy to have vaginal discharge, but I am! After using vaginal hormone cream, I am now starting to produce some fluid down there. What a bizarre thing to be happy about.

♀ My doctor put me on a vaginal hormone cream. Not only did my vaginal dryness get better, but my libido improved. It is a really good combination! I'm not sure if it is because of the hormones or just the moisture, but I'll take it either way.

What to Try: To Adjust to Surprising Physical Changes

✓ Try different moisturizers, lotions, creams and makeup to find what works best for the new characteristics of your skin.

✓ Get a facial and have an expert help you figure out exactly what your skin needs.

✓ Professionals who provide facials and waxing can become your new best friends. It might be worth it to invest in professional help so you feel better about yourself, have longer-term results than you would with do-it-yourself treatments, and get to feel pampered and relaxed.

✓ Ask your girlfriends what has worked and not worked for them.

✓ Before slathering on lotion to get rid of dry, dead skin, use a loofah or body scrub lotion to exfoliate first.

✓ Go to an upscale department store or lingerie store and get a real bra fitting and then invest in at least one really good, really comfy bra.

✓ Increase the amount of fish oils you get, either through eating more fish and/or through taking supplements. The oil can help your skin be more supple and young looking and maybe even help with vaginal dryness. FYI – it helps with dry eyes too!

✓ Use lubricating eye drops, not eye drops to get the red out or to replace tears. After using them for a little while, you just might find that not only will your eyes feel better, but you also might actually see better. If over the counter options don't work, check with a medical professional for prescription options.

✓ Try an over-the-counter vaginal lubricant that is just for overall moisturizing, not just sex, to help treat vaginal dryness and itching. If the first one doesn't work well, try another brand.

✓ If over the counter vaginal moisturizers don't work, check with your doctor to see if you can get a prescription for something stronger.

✓ Don't avoid getting vaginal hormone cream because you don't want to go get a pelvic exam. If you have had your annual gynecologist visit fairly recently, you might just be able to talk to the doctor or nurse over the phone to explain your symptoms and get a prescription called into the pharmacy.

✓ If you have intense vaginal itching that won't go away, you might have an infection that needs to be treated. And, don't assume it is a yeast infection, because there are other kinds of infections, too.

o o o

SECTION III

OMG!!!

Are you still there? We have dumped an awful lot on you that you might not have totally expected. Well, take a deep breath and get ready to keep going. Okay, maybe a few more deep breaths wouldn't hurt because next comes some of the most shocking physical changes that you might experience.

It's not really that these next changes are that horrible; it's just that you probably aren't expecting them at this time in your life. Additionally, it might be somewhat shocking to see how they seem to add up on top of each other. Sometimes it's just the sheer number of new bodily functions, or lack of functions, that will drive you crazy.

At the point when you discover some particularly bothersome symptom or feel you just can't cope with yet another, unpredictable change, you might decide to get some outside help. And, you should! We think that deciding to seek medical or alternative support is a great way to take control of your situation.

Each of us has to make our own decisions, based on our own bodies, our own preferences and our own experiences, though. There is no one perfect solution. There aren't even a dozen perfect solutions. That's why we won't even attempt to present solutions. We will just try to support you as you ask the questions, evaluate the options, and honor what feels right to you. Just making a choice and trying something proactive may make you feel better, even if it doesn't work the first time or, when you do find something that helps, it only helps for a while.

Chapter 4

You've Got to be Kidding Me! – *Shocking* Physical Changes

Dear Mother Nature: I had no idea how much a body could change and how fast it could happen. I am your hostage and at your mercy. I'm not sure whether I wished I had known in advance or if it's better that I didn't have a clue what was going to happen. Now that I'm in the thick of it, though, I wish it was easier to predict and understand the changes, not to mention to figure out what to do about them.

P.S.: Bite me.

We have hinted, joked, warned, and summarized. Now we are going to discuss, in rather blunt language, some rather shocking effects perimenopause can have. Please don't shoot the messenger.

Not By the Hair of My Chinny, Chin, Chin: Hair

You have probably heard about how menopausal women can experience thinning hair. Maybe you heard about the potential of growing more facial hair, either from your mother, aunt, older friend, or the many commercials about facial hair that have popped up on TV. But that is just the start of it. We have put "hair" in the section about shocking symptoms, instead of the section about what you might expect, because there are all sorts of other hair-raising experiences that can occur during perimenopause. Many will probably be rather unexpected since most women aren't terribly comfortable with pubic or breast hair, for example, being a topic of general conversation.

♀ Tweezers: my new best friend. Every morning I take my tweezers and a mirror over by the window where the sun shines in. The whisker hunt is on! I contort my face and turn every possible direction to spot those hairs that seem invisible at first glance, but when caught in the sunlight are about long enough (even though they were not there the day before) to floss your teeth with, without even pulling them out first. I feel all over my face for the now familiar prickle of new growth, checking all of the places that are becoming the usual spots, but always looking for new ones that are sprouting up with newfound regularity. Oh, and don't forget the wonderfully glamorous and special mole whiskers! They are so bristly you could clean the grill with them. Does it get any more feminine than that?

♀ If a whisker is left to its own devices for several days, you could inadvertently poke someone's eye out just by turning your head.

♀ I never understood the need for those light-up magnifying mirrors, but they seem like a brilliant invention now. You'd think whiskers were enough facial hair to deal with, but no, I also need hair removal cream for my newly expanded moustache. Those thick, bountiful hairs now cover not only the area above the lip, but are also creeping down the sides of my mouth. If this keeps up much longer, I could have a goatee. And the eyebrows? What is up with those long crazy ones that grow 3 times as long as the others and love to stand up and check out the world? I thought it was only old men and crazy uncles who had those.

♀ I thought that those hair trimmers that you stick up your nose were only for men. Nope! Now I am freaking out about my ears too. I can't see them. I am trying to figure out which girlfriend I have the guts to ask to check for me.

♀ My girlfriends and I have a pact. If any of us is in the hospital unconscious for any reason, it is the others' responsibility to bring tweezers to the hospital and take care of all stray hairs. It is our version of a living will.

♀ Sitting at a street light in my car is my time to feel all over my face to find new whiskers that have appeared. I am sure people in other cars wonder what the heck I am doing. I wonder what they will think when I pull out the tweezers and start working on them! That is the next step!

♀ I no longer have to worry about how skimpy my eyelashes are. I'll just stop plucking my eyebrows for a few days and let them fill in my entire eyelid.

♀ The hair is thinning on the top of my head at the same time my nostril hairs, ear hairs, chin hairs, upper lip hairs, and pubic hairs are going into overdrive. I'm afraid to take any of those hair growth medications to improve the hair on my head because I'm afraid I'll end up a bald gorilla.

♀ It's bad enough that I have stiff, dark whisker hairs sticking out here and there on my chin, but in between and all over my cheeks I have peach fuzz. It is so pale that when the sun catches it, I look fuzzy. Am I supposed to wax or use hair-removing cream all over my face?

♀ OMG! I found a whisker on my nipple!

♀ I think I am getting peach fuzz on my chest and belly as well as on my cheeks. I am going to dunk myself in a vat of hair removal cream soon.

♀ "Has your hair been this fly-away lately?" my hair stylist of over 20 years asked me. Actually, it had, I admitted. She asked what shampoo I had been using. "The one you recommended to me over 10 years ago," I replied. "Well," she said with a shrug, "you need a moisturizing shampoo now." Unbelievable. The hair on my head is getting dry, too! I guess it wants to keep my vagina company.

♀ The one good thing about getting gray like I am is that I don't have to pay for highlights anymore. When I color my hair, the grey naturally comes out a lighter color. Celebrate the little victories!

♀ There is one very stubborn gray pubic hair that is right in the middle where it is very visible. I keep pulling it out, but it grows right back. It is really getting to be a pain because now that my belly is all bloated and saggy, I sort of have to move it out of the way to be able to look down and see the damn hair to pluck it out!

♀ I had heard about thinning hair as something that sometimes happens to middle-aged women. I thought that losing some thickness in my hair wouldn't be such a bad thing. I didn't realize that it is more like male balding where you can get really thin in certain places on the scalp. Where I part my hair is getting wider and wider.

♀ I am thinking of taking a hair loss product, despite the potential side effects. I see more and more hair in the sink and the shower drain over time. I can handle a lot of things but losing my hair isn't one of them.

♀ I am convinced my hair is migrating toward my middle. The hair on my head seems to be moving down onto my face. The hair on my shins is

57

moving up to my thighs and belly. Do you think I could get a pubic hair transplant and put it up on my head? I can just picture the doctor's face when I ask for that!

♀ Brazilian wax, my ass (literally)! I need all of South America waxed at this point!

♀ I know it is called pubic hair, but I have taken to calling it "public" hair since it is growing out of bounds and is thicker than ever. I have to shave every day during the summer or shorts and bathing suits are definitely off limits.

♀ Pubic hair can now be measured in square footage and seems longer than the hair on my head. Unreal. I actually have to cut the hair because it gets so long.

♀ I try to avoid looking at my stomach these days, but something caught my eye in the mirror the other day. I have hair now all the way up from my pubic area to my belly button! And, I am not talking about just a few hairs. Gee, just when I thought I couldn't feel less sexy. My husband calls it the "stairway to heaven," which makes it a little better.

♀ When I first started having perimenopausal symptoms, it seemed like I had more pubic hair. Now that I hardly ever have a period anymore, it seems like it has not only gone back to normal, but maybe even less than normal. I would not be the least bit unhappy to have less hair to shave at the bikini line!

♀ The farther apart my periods get, the less hairy my legs and armpits seem to be. I still have to pluck my eyebrows every other day, but at least I don't seem to need to shave quite so often. Of course, in actuality, it might be that I either don't see or don't care about the hair on my legs or under my arms as much as I used to, but either way, I don't have to deal with it as much anymore!

Turn the Other Cheek: Butt and Bowels

"Rectum??? Darn near killed 'em!!" Sorry, we just couldn't help ourselves. (Say it out loud if you don't get it right away.) Buttocks and rectums are no more subjects for polite conversation than are vaginas. So, of course, it's appropriate to talk about them here!

As if just discussing flabby asses isn't uncomfortable enough, let's throw constipation and hemorrhoids into the pot (pun intended). It's not fun to think about, but constipation and hemorrhoids, as well as anal itching and anal fissures, are anything but unusual for women during perimenopause. And men wonder why we are never in the mood.

♀ The other night I thought I got my period after using the restroom and seeing quite a bit of blood in the toilet. Well, guess what? It was coming from my rectum, not my vagina. Turns out I have an anal fissure which is "common for women my age." I have prescription butt cream now. Oh, joy.

♀ I am hearing about more and more women my age suffering from hemorrhoids so bad they need surgery or medical intervention. I wonder if it is because so many of us are constipated. Or maybe it is because things internally are sagging as much as things externally.

♀ I have literally switched to a softer toilet paper because wiping can be such agony these days.

♀ My pubic hair used to stay in my pubic region. Now it is growing up my crack.

♀ I thought pelvic exams couldn't get any worse, but the last time I went for my annual gyno appointment, he did a rectal exam for the first time. This is just another one of the fun joys of this stage of life, I guess. It's not painful, but it is a very strange feeling.

♀ Having a bowel movement is cause for a big celebration these days. Something that I never used to have to even think about now preoccupies my mind. I get so bloated and uncomfortable, but I am lucky if I go twice a week.

♀ Fiber – it's not just for old people anymore! MiraLAX® and FiberCon® and Citrucel®, oh my! Whatever your regimen needs to be, just get it done! It makes such a difference. Who knew that the poop was just supposed to slide out with such little fuss? And, in one piece, as opposed to 10 hard little balls?

♀ My husband doesn't think it is nearly as funny as I do when I come out of the bathroom after a big poop, throw my arms in the air like a referee after a field goal and yell, "score!" My girlfriends get it, though.

♀ Is being gassy related to perimenopause? Is nothing sacred?

♀ Everyone farts, but in the past, mine have always been quiet and lady-like. There are times now when I sound like a truck-driver. Worst of all, sometimes I can't even hold it in until I can get to a safe place. This is my most embarrassing perimenopausal symptom.

♀ Is an itchy butt a perimenopausal symptom? Funny, I've never heard anyone talk about it. I hope that if I am brave enough to say something, though, other women will say they have experienced the same thing, too.

♀ My ass seems to be sliding down the back of my thighs. No matter how hard I exercise, I just can't get it to firm up and lift up. Foundation undergarments seem to be in my not-too-distant future.

♀ I took a few minutes the other day to really look at my rear in the mirror. To my total dismay, it was a total stranger, nothing like I remember it looking in days gone by. It is flat, long, wide, and my cheeks rest on the backs of my thighs. The skin is not milky and smooth anymore like I remember it. It's more like the skin of an old, over-ripe orange.

Not Tonight, Honey: Headaches

Who ever heard about headaches being part of perimenopause? It turns out that some women report an increase in headaches. Others report a decrease. Some get migraines. Some with migraines get fewer. Do we need to say it again? You just never know.

♀ I have always struggled with migraines, but since I have been in perimenopause, they have become less frequent, but way more intense. I was ready to go to the hospital the last one was so bad.

♀ I feel like my head is buzzing sometimes. It's not really a headache, but not really my ears ringing, either.

♀ It was common for me to get headaches as part of my PMS. Now that I seem to be getting PMS at strange times and for longer periods (ha!), it seems like I am getting more headaches, too.

♀ My head sometimes aches, but it isn't what I would normally consider a headache. I sort of wonder if it isn't just the side effects of too little sleep and too much trouble seeing.

♀ It would be really nice to be able to drown my sorrows in a few drinks, but that only makes things worse. The least little bit of alcohol seems to give me a headache these days. It's like getting a hangover when I haven't had anything close to what it would have taken to give me a hangover in the past.

♀ Perimenopause is a headache in and of itself. I am not sure if it is actual hormone changes or just the stress and tension from the hormone changes, but I get headaches much more frequently than I used to.

♀ I have discovered that some of my headaches are actually from tension in my neck. The tension in my neck could be because I am not sleeping well, feel like I have turned into a raving lunatic, or any of the many other symptoms I have been experiencing. Who knows? What I do know is that occasionally getting a massage is really helping not only my headaches, but my all-over tension.

Ain't No Body I Know: General Physical Changes

We have tried to list as many of the expected, surprising, and shocking physical symptoms of this stage of life as possible in the previous chapters, but we wouldn't want to make it sound like there is a checklist. Some women will experience lots of symptoms related to hair and practically none related to body shape, for example. Others will have a little of everything.

Unfortunately, there is no way to predict exactly what your particular experience will be like, how intense your symptoms will be, or how long it will last. One way to find out what you're likely to experience is to talk to your mom, since you will likely follow a similar pattern. Of course, nothing is certain with perimenopause, so we are providing the following stories that give some examples of what other women have experienced overall.

♀ I had my "annual" exam today. Typically, it includes some chit-chat, a Pap, a breast exam, and I am on my way. Not the case today. I spent over 30 minutes with my doctor and left with the following:

- A prescription for an antidepressant that supposedly is great for "women my age" and the crazy things that are happening to my body and mind.
- Believe it or not, a prescription for birth control pills even though I've had my tubes tied. I guess for women in their 40's who are still having periods they can be very helpful with the symptoms that are caused by low estrogen. Please, God.
- Prenatal vitamins (apparently they will help me feel better too).
- A prescription for a stool softener to "get things going" and directions for daily use of flax seed oil and FiberCon®. I guess it is not normal to only poop once a week. Who knew?
- A prescription for cholesterol medication as my cholesterol is skyrocketing with this newfound poundage that has glommed onto my body.
- A prescription for a yeast infection – I thought all that fun itching was from dryness.
- An order for a mammogram.
- An order for blood work to get a baseline of my hormone levels.

Oh, and I got a flu shot while I was at it. I did get the Pap smear and breast exam. I have never felt so old and so unhealthy in my life.

♀ Rather than worry about what my hormone levels indicate about where I am in the aging process, I am measuring my way through perimenopause and my 40's based on the number of medicine bottles in my bathroom. It started with the basics: Tylenol® and multi-vitamins. Additional supplements soon followed. Then it was medication for Gastric Reflux Disease. High cholesterol medication, medication for bladder control, and antidepressants soon followed. Now, I am starting a variety of homeopathic creams and pills to try to control the hot flashes. I can't believe this is happening so early. Is it just because we see all the medication ads on TV, because there are so many more tests, or because we are identifying and dealing with health issues much earlier than we used to? I wasn't expecting it to be like this until I was in my 60's at least. I am giving my grandmother a run for her money in the race for who is taking the most medications!

♀ On top of all the irritating hormone-related physical symptoms I am experiencing, there also seem to be a lot of changes that just relate to getting older. I wish it was just one or the other. I hate having turned into what feels like an old lady. I am dry, losing hair, and have to pick up a toothpick after a meal with all the old fogies. My nose runs, so I keep a Kleenex tucked in my bag at all times. Hell, I am the old bag!

♀ It's scary to think that one day I will look back on the body I have today and wish I had appreciated it more. All I can see right now is the thickening around the middle that I can't control, the wrinkles around my eyes, and my sagging jowls. I think back to the body I had when I was 30 and wish I had been more daring, more showy, more dramatic, and more grateful for what I had then.

♀ Recently I have noticed a "pooch" that seems impossible to get rid of. Even participating in a near starvation diet doesn't help. Plus, I pee a bit when I laugh or sneeze. I've taken to wearing a mini-pad sometimes! My husband is always wondering why I wear a pad. When I finally told him I may pee on myself, it quickly ended the conversation!

♀ Everything is migrating toward my middle. The hair on my head and shins is getting thinner while I am getting more hair on my thighs, stomach, and chin. My shoulders, boobs, and the skin on my face are all sagging. My butt is sagging down more, but it has lost the volume that my hips seem to have gained. My waist is getting thicker and thicker even though I haven't gained weight. I am going to look like Violet Beauregard did when she blew up into a blueberry and got rolled away in the movie *Charlie and the Chocolate Factory*.

♀ I have to be so careful of what I wear for so many reasons. Light colored pants or skirts scare me because I might leak through. Dark colored clothes are dangerous because they end up covered in flakes of dry skin. Everything I own feels tight around the waist. Anything with the tiniest bit of wool or rough seams is a no-no because I will be itchy all over.

♀ You know how the Pillsbury Doughboy™ looks? That's how I feel. Even when I exercise, my body does not feel as toned as it used to be.

♀ I've never had to use deodorant. As my hormones started to change, though, I realized that I had body odor and had to start using it. It's not any big deal, just one more strange change.

♀ Just like when I was pregnant, I am so sensitive to smells now. One of my friends commented on how often I have been mentioning how things smell. I don't remember ever doing that except when I was pregnant.

♀ How weird is it that my perfume, which I have used for years, just doesn't smell the same on me anymore. I thought maybe it was just my sense of smell changing, but I asked my friend and she agreed it seemed different now. It must be reacting with my hormones differently. Or, rather, my different hormones are reacting with it differently.

♀ My body is like the Sahara desert. I am dry everywhere. My hair, my skin, my vagina, my mouth, my eyes – all dry, dry, dry.

♀ It seems like I had a stress-induced mini-menopause. During a time of extreme work pressure, my periods slowed down to virtually nothing, I got pretty depressed, and I had a variety of perimenopause symptoms, like hot flashes. Then, as things calmed down, I started feeling tons better. My periods were still irregular, I was still growing a few hairs on my chin that hadn't been there before, and I was a bit more melancholy than usual, but things were much, much better. I am hoping that this little trial period will make it easier to go through it for real the next time. Or, maybe I will have gone through the worst of it already.

♀ After 45 days without a period and feeling very strange, I took a pregnancy test. At 42, I hoped to God that it was negative. It was. Ten days later, no period and more strange symptoms. Another negative pregnancy test. Hmmmm ... Could something else be going on? Finally, a period. Okay, back on track for a few months. Then, another 60 days or so without a period and feeling very weird. Another pregnancy test. Then, duh, the light went off. Could this be the beginning of menopause? For 2 years, I fluctuated between perfectly normal, but really light periods for several months, then a few months of skipped periods. Then, during a period of very intense stress in my life, I got almost all of the symptoms that I now know to associate with perimenopause. Okay, I thought. If this is it, bring it on so I can get it over with sooner. Just as I got used to the idea, I had a few months of semi-normal periods. Now that my stress level has gone down, I still have some symptoms, but not so many. I still fluctuate a lot and skip periods more and more. I have no idea what will come next, but I have invested heavily in mini-pads, super maxi-pads, tweezers, vaginal lubricant, reading glasses, and sticky notes. I am ready for anything!

♀ When will I feel like I understand and can predict my body again? 'Round and 'round she goes. Where she stops, nobody knows!

♀ Now I understand yet another reason why it is good to start getting regular physicals at this age. I found out that hormone changes can even affect my cholesterol level. Is there anything at all that it doesn't affect? Or, is it just that as we age these things naturally happen and in women, it is blamed on hormones. Either way, I feel like I just suddenly became my parents, sitting around talking to their friends about all their medical problems.

♀ I get a magazine that is designed just for women in this stage of life. I really love it. I wonder, though, as I look at the famous women who are my age or older but who look decades younger, if this magazine does a little airbrushing or if those women are just incredibly lucky genetically and/or have amazing makeup artists. What does it say if even magazines for women in their 40's and 50's feel the need to hide crow's feet, wrinkly skin, and a little sagging around the jaw line? I'd just love for the magazine to do a spread and show these women without makeup and in normal clothes to see if they look their true ages in real life.

♀ I have all the usual suspects for what I used to think was "early" menopause (now I know it is perimenopause): irregular periods, occasional hot flashes, changes in my skin tone, and the feeling that my mind just isn't quite right. What bothers me the most, though, is just the vague sense of discomfort. No matter how much I sleep, I am tired. No matter how much I exercise, I don't quite feel in shape. I just don't feel right, and nothing I do seems to help me feel like I used to.

♀ I had never heard about sore joints being related to hormonal fluctuations. When I mentioned that my joints have been aching for no reason, though, a few of my girlfriends mentioned that they were having the same thing. When I researched it, I found that this is a known, but not often mentioned, symptom of perimenopause. Gee, I guess this is preparing me for arthritis.

♀ In the last few months, I have had to start being careful about what lotions, makeup, laundry detergent, and other products I use. I get rashes and allergic reactions much more easily than I used to.

What to Try: To Adjust to Shocking Physical Changes

✓ Buy a really good pair of tweezers, a magnifying mirror with a strong light, hair removal cream, and whatever else you need to deal with facial hair.

✓ Switch to hair care products that are suited for the new needs of your hair. You might need shampoo that is extra moisturizing or designed to create extra volume for example. You might want to switch the types of gels or sprays you use, too. Talk to your hair stylist to see what she recommends.

✓ Now might be a good time to try professional hair removal for stubborn whiskers on your chin, nipples, belly, or other bothersome areas.

✓ Use hair removal products only on the body parts for which they are designed. Some skin, such as your nipples, may be too sensitive for harsh chemicals.

✓ Butts don't change for the better on their own. Try new exercises that target the danger zones.

✓ If you are experiencing rectal bleeding, get it checked out. Most internists or family practitioners are qualified to do a basic check for hemorrhoids and can even handle some of the basic treatments. If things are more complicated, you might get referred for an exam by a specialist or a colonoscopy. You know you are going to have to have a colonoscopy anyway within the upcoming years. Why put it off if there is something that could be caught early?

✓ We picked the right time to get flabby bellies and saggy butts. There is a wide variety of shaping garments available these days. If you hate how you look in clothes, try them out.

✓ Some department stores have free personal shoppers who can help you figure out what styles will look best on you now. Getting some professional help can make you feel a lot better about yourself.

✓ Try to find a friend with whom you feel comfortable discussing the changes that bother or scare you. It can really help to talk out loud about these things. Usually, you will find that you are perfectly normal, even if they were shocking to you. And, if what you are experiencing isn't normal, it's good to know that, too, so you can do something about it.

○ ○ ○

Chapter 5

To Hormone or Not to Hormone, That is the Question – Perimenopausal Treatment

Dear Mother Nature: Maybe I could beat you at your own game and replace the hormones you have taken away. I'll show you! Although . . . can I even do it now since I still have some periods? Are the trade-offs worth it? Are there side effects? Will I only be getting rid of some annoying problems that aren't really affecting my health? Will I have new problems? Will it negatively affect my health or even cause cancer? Everyone I talk to has a different opinion.

PS: Wishin' I were a man right now.

How do you treat the symptoms? Hormones, homeopathics, supplements, soy? What are your preferences in general when it comes to medical versus alternative therapies? It is good to think about these types of questions (whenever your mind feels clear enough).

Many of us believe that there are things, such as taking hormones, which we will *never* do. Most of us have a symptom that is our biggest fear and worry. Unfortunately, sometimes those two things clash. When faced with a truly intolerable experience, your thoughts about what you will *never* do might just change. There is nothing wrong with that, though.

During perimenopause, like during childbirth, there is no way to know what you will feel, how your body will react, and what all your choices will be until you are in the midst of it. Many a pregnant women, for example, went into labor thinking that she absolutely would go natural no matter what and that medical interventions would take her control away and ruin the experience. Then she found that the pain, the desire to make the best choice for her baby, or the feeling that she was losing control meant changing her mind and getting an epidural or other intervention. Sometimes, when your body truly feels horrible, the bad physical stuff gets in the way of the good mental stuff. Taking away some of the physical symptoms can help your mind function better. Then, you can enjoy the experience and be happier, even if you end up doing something differently than you originally expected.

We encourage you to research your options, keep your mind open, and constantly re-evaluate your choices. This is the best way for you to feel in control because you will always be the decision-maker, always be the one prioritizing your issues. When your body feels so wacky, it will feel good to have some sense of control over how you are handling it, even if you can't completely manage how your body reacts.

Doctor, Doctor Give me a Clue: Getting Medical Support

This is not a time of life when you want to rely just on the medical information you can find online. It can be helpful, but it isn't enough. Whether you want to use a medical professional just for the basics at your annual visit or more aggressively to help address your perimenopausal symptoms, it's important to have a relationship in which you feel comfortable openly discussing anything that is bothering you.

If your medical professional's approach to managing perimenopause doesn't match yours, go find someone who is a better fit. Talk to your girlfriends, talk to your other doctors, or go online to check out Web sites to get referral information. Do the best you can to find a supportive medical relationship *before* you are in a difficult or upsetting situation.

♀ After months of feeling like I must be horribly ill, I finally talked to my doctor about all the strange things I had been experiencing. After doing my full annual exam, he assured me that nothing was wrong other than that I was in perimenopause. At first I was relieved and happy about that. Then I did a bit of research and realized that this wasn't going to be any party, either!

♀ I don't know or care specifically what my hormones are doing. When I ask my doctor about menopause, I don't want to hear about the scientific explanation of menopause. I want to know if what I am experiencing is normal for this stage of my life and hormones, what I should expect, and what my options are. And, I want my doctor to take the time and energy to explore my choices with me.

♀ We don't "treat" puberty or pregnancy. Why does my doctor talk about "treating" my perimenopause symptoms? I am not sick. I just

70

want to cope with it better. I try to explain the difference to him, but he just doesn't get it.

♀ My doctor told me my body is in a race. My uterine fibroids are growing so fast that they are starting to push on other organs. He said that maybe I will go into menopause soon enough that they will shrink due to the reduction in estrogen. Am I supposed to think that this is a good thing? Will I be winning the race or losing?

♀ I have been asking my doctor for years to check my hormones. He keeps telling me that I am too young, that knowing my hormone levels won't change anything. I just want to know! Am I in the beginning, middle or near the end of this process? He may not care, but I do. I am switching to a doctor who has been really supportive of one of my friends. My current doctor was great when I was having kids and dealing with birth control, but he is not at all sympathetic or helpful now. Time to switch to a middle-aged female doc!

♀ It's corny, but my favorite joke these days is, "How do you make a hormone? Don't pay her." Say it out loud if you don't get it.

♀ I don't think anyone understands how hormones work or how to replace them. They try, but no one really knows how. I am very uncomfortable feeling like a guinea pig, trying one thing after another without any real sense of what will work or what is safe for long-term health.

♀ If men had to go through perimenopause, you'd better believe there would be a test to find out how far along you are in the process. Hell, they would have figured out to make self-regulating hormone pills a long time ago. There are tests for almost everything else these days, why isn't there a test for this?

♀ So what if my hormones are fluctuating over time, from day to day and month-to-month. Couldn't I get tested over time to see what is going on? I know my insurance wouldn't pay for it (even though it did pay when my husband's testosterone level was checked as part of a normal physical!), but I would pay out of pocket if necessary. It seems to me that having a baseline level would help figure out how far along I am in the process. How can hormones be prescribed to replace my missing hormones if they have no idea how much I am missing?

♀ My middle-aged male OB/GYN is missing the point. Because he is also getting wrinkly, losing his eyesight, and gaining weight, he likes to tell me that everything I am going through is just due to age, not hormones. Of course, in the past when I mentioned PMS or pregnancy symptoms that were bothering me, it was all about hormones! Why has that suddenly changed? I think it is because he just doesn't know what to do and has a handy response that will shut me down. Very frustrating. Time for a new doctor!

♀ I have found that my regular internist doctor is very helpful when it comes to discussing my current symptoms and frustrations. Since things seem to be changing so much and I tend to see my regular doctor more often, it's nice not to have to wait to talk with my gynecologist once a year or to schedule an additional appointment with her.

♀ One of my friends gave me the best advice ever when I got frustrated because my doctor just didn't seem to be taking my symptoms seriously. She said that I should make a daily list of all the things in my life that frustrate me, not just my physical symptoms. When I went down that list with my doctor, I didn't say that I was really tired. I told him the truth about how I just couldn't summon the energy to get out of bed on some days. He realized that I was depressed and he even believed that I was having perimenopause symptoms that needed to be treated. After only a few months of treatment for the depression, I felt a lot better. The perimenopause symptoms got much better, too.

You Can't Always Get What You Want: Evaluating Your Choices

The good news is that there are tons of choices for addressing the various aspects of perimenopause. The bad news is that there are tons of choices for addressing the various aspects of perimenopause.

♀ I am aware that there are a variety of hormone treatments available for menopausal symptoms. What frustrates me is that it seems like so many of the side effects are as bad as or worse than what they supposedly treat. I might be able to avoid drying up, but I could gain weight. I can minimize the problems associated with lower estrogen, but I might increase my chances of some types of cancer. I also don't really understand when I am supposed to go on them. I still have my period, although it is very irregular. Do I start hormones now or wait until they are all gone and I am post-menopausal?

♀ What's the first thing you do when you want to research something these days? Go to the Internet, of course. But, if you go to the Internet to research menopause, the information is incredibly unclear. Some resources discuss premenopause; some mention perimenopause. Some talk about menopause as if it is a long period of time; others make it sound like the point at which you haven't had a period for twelve months, after which you are post-menopausal. The information is confusing because the labels aren't consistent. Do women like me, with irregular periods and lots of symptoms like hot flashes, itchy skin, and vaginal dryness, get to take hormones or would that cause cancer? It really pisses me off that it is so hard to get consistent, helpful information. My doctor isn't even that helpful.

♀ Not only can't I carefully evaluate my options, but I'm having trouble even determining what my options are! It seems like every few years the medical experts change their minds about what does or doesn't cause cancer. For every article about the benefits of herbs, there is another one describing the risks, for example. And, since the information isn't terribly clear about what can be used when you're still getting periods occasionally, it is difficult to determine what options are available during perimenopause, not just after menopause.

♀ Do I give up something that makes me feel better but creates a different but minor problem? It seems that no matter what choices I make, there is always a side effect to consider.

♀ The instructions on a jar of progesterone cream from the health food store say to do one thing if you are premenopausal and another if you are menopausal or post-menopausal. What am I if I got my last period 7 months ago?

♀ It seems like every time I go to the vitamin or health food store, the section that has women's menopause therapies gets bigger and bigger. It's nice to have all those choices, but it also means that there are so many to choose from without a whole lot of info on what works best in which situations. And, they aren't cheap!

♀ If one more article tells me to eat right, exercise, and cut down the stress in my life, I will scream! Haven't they been telling us that for years? How exactly is that supposed to help perimenopause symptoms in particular? I think it is just a general catch-all solution when they don't know what else to tell us.

♀ I am shocked at how many different options there are out there for almost every perimenopausal symptom. Some make sense. Others seem crazy. I wish there was more information out there from reliable sources about what works and what doesn't. Isn't anyone tracking the trends in what works and what doesn't?

♀ *Fried Green Tomatoes* has always been one of my favorite movies. Last night I was flipping channels and caught the second half of it. I have loved that movie for years but until I saw it this time, I never realized how much of Evelyn's (Kathy Bates) character is based on her being in perimenopause. At one point, she is complaining about her frustrations to her new friend, Ms. Threadgood (Jessica Tandy), saying how she can't stand her husband, can't lose weight, and is "too young to be old and too old to be young." The older, wiser character comforts her by saying something along the lines of, "Why, dear, you're going through the change. You need to get yourself some of them hormones!" Evelyn looks at her in total shock as if that thought had never occurred to her, but she is thrilled there is a reason for how she's feeling and a potential solution. Later in the movie, when Evelyn has started paying attention to herself instead of her husband and is explaining how excited she is to feel like she is taking her own life in her hands for the first time (including bashing in the back-end of a car after two young girls stole the parking space she was waiting for), Ms. Threadgood says, "Honey, just how many of those hormones are you takin'?" Seeing this movie while I am in this stage of life let me see a whole new aspect to the story that I had totally missed before! It was great to be reminded about how many generations of women have gone through these same frustrations and had to decide how they are going to get through them. It was also a good reminder that sometimes we just need to open up to someone and let them help point us in the right direction before we can open our eyes to our options.

♀ Thank goodness for the Internet. There is a wealth of information about there. I find that the best strategy for me is first to research well-respected sites from places like the Mayo clinic. That usually leads me to a few terms or concepts that I'd like to research more. Then I'll look for those terms or concepts on Web sites from women's menopause groups. Then I go to chat rooms and read what other women write. I feel like this gives me a good sense of what to believe versus what are personal perspectives. I have yet to write my own feelings, but it's nice to know I could if I wanted to.

♀ I am tired of talking about my options when my feet are up in the air and the doctor is between my legs. I set up a separate appointment that didn't include an exam so we could just talk about how everything else besides my vagina feels and what I can do about it.

♀ It's amazing what a help girlfriends can be. You might never know someone has been going through something difficult or has tried a certain therapy unless you bring it up in conversation. Now I have started talking more about what I'm going through. I have learned some very helpful information and found out about options that I would never have known about otherwise.

Eeny, Meeny, Miney, Moe: Deciding What is Right for You

Managing perimenopausal symptoms is not an exact science. There is no one "right" way or plan. Just as we are all shaped differently, have different symptoms (and to varying degrees), and react differently to medication, we each have to find what is uniquely "right" for ourselves.

If at first you don't succeed, try, try again. Even if you do succeed, what's right for you today might not be right for you tomorrow, next week, or next year. Even if you feel really good about your current choices, there might be more decisions for you to make in the future as your body continues to change. Rather than beating yourself up for making a choice that didn't continue to be right, give yourself permission to make another decision whenever necessary.

♀ I choose to do only those things that can easily be integrated into my normal lifestyle. My treatment plan is more exercise, less stress (or at least relaxation time to cope with the stress), lots of veggies, cutting down on soda and drinking more milk, taking calcium supplements, and generally just trying to be healthier – all the things I always said I should do, I finally am doing. I feel the difference, too!

♀ Why in the world wouldn't I use a treatment that is available to get rid of all these horrible symptoms?

♀ My mother thinks I am crazy for wanting to avoid hormones. She says that in her day, women looked forward to it. I am just so nervous about how every few years the medical experts seem to find new information that says what had been the magic pill a few years earlier is now known to cause cancer. I doubt natural hormone changes alone cause cancer, so my instinct is to just bully my way through all this without taking anything.

♀ For some reason, I am very, very reluctant to treat what are essentially natural physical changes with formal Western medicine. I don't have any problem using prescription medication when I have an infection or a disease, but somehow this situation feels different. I want to try alternative, more natural approaches first and see what happens.

♀ Right now I can deal with the perimenopause symptoms naturally. I think I will even do alternative therapies to deal with the potential of heart disease and bone loss. I will do it as long as possible, but if they don't work, I will switch to more formal medical approaches. In other words, I will do the best of both worlds.

♀ My doctor said that it is a good thing that I have a few extra pounds since the fat carries estrogen in it. Unreal. I can't believe that during this stage one of the worst things about my body turns into a good thing! He told me that I would probably do better through perimenopause if I don't diet to lose weight, but just try to eat healthier. I have given myself permission not to get so upset about the extra weight.

♀ It seems like the recommended hormone therapy changes every few years as more long-term data comes in. Whatever I decide to do, I will do it in moderation with the lowest possible doses, careful monitoring, and the shortest time period possible. I will also wait as long as possible before making the final decision about whether or not to use hormones.

♀ I can't decide whether I am more afraid of future heart disease and osteoporosis or current mental lapses, constant irritability, and gushing periods.

♀ I've been having symptoms for several years and told myself that at some point they would be bad enough to treat. I just keep redefining what "bad enough" is. Of course, I also have to consider the flip side. As if the hot flashes, dryness, and crazy periods aren't enough, what is happening to my bones? I feel like I should take that into consideration too, but I just can't figure out what the "right" thing is to do.

♀ I try not to worry about what may happen in the distant future. I am more concerned with feeling good now!

♀ I am careful about what I eat. I regularly do yoga and Pilates. I get plenty of rest, and I drink a lot of water. Whenever possible, I go to a holistic practitioner rather than a medical doctor. I take supplements. I live as natural and healthy a life as I can. I just have not been able to find anything that treats my lack of sex drive, my intensely dry skin, and my wicked hot flashes. I finally decided to try the hormones my doctor has offered. I feel soooo much better. I will continue to do everything else as naturally as possible, but I will not give up the hormones. They made me feel like me again.

♀ I resorted to taking birth control pills, which I have never taken before, while I was in perimenopause. I try to do everything naturally and really didn't want to have to do it, but I just felt horrible and couldn't find anything else that helped. Once I started, everything felt better. My skin wasn't so dry and saggy, my mood was better, and I could think again. I compare the decision to use hormones to the decision to get an epidural during labor. I really wanted to go all natural, but I just had no idea how hard it was going to be. Before it was real, it was easy to think that I was going to be strong enough to get through it alone. In both cases, I was really glad there were medical options that could help me during a really difficult time.

♀ I don't have a hard time with the idea of using hormones to get through a few years of difficult menopause-related symptoms, but I can't stand the idea of staying on them forever. My doctor seems to think that it isn't a problem, but I just hate the idea. Of course, I also worry about having the same symptoms again if I do decide to go off them in the future. Maybe by that time, there will be some other alternatives available.

♀ I am totally comfortable going on birth control pills as a hormone treatment while I am in perimenopause. I am even happy to go on hormones when I am in menopause, but how will I know when to go off them? My mother has been on them for 30 years. She says she will never go off them, no matter what!

♀ My small, thin body type leads me to believe that I could be the "poster child" for osteoporosis, but I hope to offset problems by continuing to exercise and eat correctly. Even though I have a "plan," it's still tough to get those physical cues that make me feel like I am focusing on the negatives versus the positive. My attitude will affect those around me, though, so I plan to fight the emotions as best as I can.

♀ I have started a journal so I can keep track of when I start to notice a symptom, how it develops, what methods I have tried to control them, what results I have gotten, and any other pertinent info. Otherwise, I lose track of what is or isn't working. It also helps me identify when I feel ready to wean off something that has worked to see if the symptoms would still be there. It is sort of a pain, but it also helps me feel in control, like I am actively managing what is going on rather than just reacting.

What to Try: To Deal with Perimenopausal Symptoms

✓ Trying to cope with each and every symptom you are experiencing could turn into a full-time and very frustrating job. Instead, identify a few symptoms that bother you the most and focus on them. If you can find a way to make them better, then you can move on to the next few. This approach can keep you from getting overwhelmed and help you gain a sense of control over what is going on with your body.

✓ Keep a record of when your periods start, how long they last, and how heavy they are so your doctor can see patterns and so you can remember. It would be a damn shame to actually get out of the perimenopause stage and into the menopause stage and not even know it!

✓ Ask about your doctor's philosophy on "treating" the symptoms of perimenopause or menopause. If he/she is adamantly pro- or anti-hormone therapy or pro- or anti-alternative therapy, it is good to know before you start discussing your personal options and preferences.

✓ Even if you are fairly sure symptoms such as heart palpitations or headaches are related to your stage of life, it is still a good thing to mention them to a doctor just in case they could be signs of something else.

✓ If you know your female family's history with respect to menopause and some of the medical side effects of loss of estrogen, like osteoporosis, share it with your doctor. It might help predict what your experience will be like or how you might react to certain therapies.

✓ If the doctor promotes use of any type of hormones (including birth control pills and hormone creams) here are things to ask:

- When does she suggest starting them and what symptoms are the key indicators for their use?
- Does she prescribe them for every perimenopausal woman or just some? If for just some, why does she recommend them for you in particular?
- How long does she suggest staying on them?
- What are the indicators or side effects that mean you should consider discontinuing them?
- How does she manage or avoid other health risks, such as breast or uterine cancer, related to use of hormones?
- What monitoring is done while you are on hormones?
- What hormone options are available, and what are their pros and cons?

✓ If you aren't comfortable discussing your concerns with your doctor, either psych yourself up to do it even though it makes you uncomfortable or find a doctor with whom you are comfortable talking openly.

79

✓ If you are trying lots of different treatments, keep a log to track when you made changes, what you changed, what new symptoms popped up, what old symptoms went away or got better. When you and/or your doctor go over your notes, trends and patterns might become obvious that you wouldn't otherwise have been able to identify. This can help you figure out what is working and what isn't.

✓ When you start a new medication, make sure to keep track of what improves, what doesn't improve and what gets worse – both physically and emotionally. Since we are dealing with hormones here, both are important and both can be affected dramatically. Only you can determine what you are and aren't willing to tolerate, but the only way you can make a good decision is to be as aware as possible of *all* the changes. Then, if something isn't working out for you, make sure to discuss it with your doctor. Sometimes a change in dosage will make a difference. Sometimes it will be better to switch to something different.

✓ Remember, your hormone levels are changing over time, so how you deal with them (or without them, as the case may be) will likely change over time.

✓ If you want to consider the various types of homeopathic, alternative therapies, it's best to get some assistance from an expert, just as you should if you choose a more traditional medical approach. A good place to start is a respected health food or vitamin store. There are also homeopathic practitioners. The best way to find good ones is to network with your friends who use these types of therapies.

✓ If you experience mood swings, depression, and/or anxiety that seriously interferes with your ability to function, talk to your doctor about medication such as antidepressants. Sometimes they can even make you feel better physically as well as resolve emotional struggles.

✓ Don't attribute absolutely everything to perimenopause. If something is unusual, making you worry, or getting significantly worse, talk with your medical professional to make sure there isn't something else going on.

Please note: As brilliant as we think the advice in this book is, please do not rely on it for medical guidance!

o   o   o

○　○　○

SECTION IV

MIND GAMES

These days, it seems that as our waists expand, our minds waste away. A mind is a terrible thing to waste, as the saying goes. It's not even the forgetfulness, though, which was somewhat expected (although at a much later date). We could excuse that because of the busyness in our lives. It's also a seeming inability to get our brains to function normally on any regular basis. Worse, it's not just that we occasionally find ourselves pulling a total blank in the middle of a very important meeting or forgetting how to get to a friend's house. It's that sometimes we just don't feel like ourselves. The things we used to like aren't the things we like now. The ways we used to mentally approach our lives just aren't working.

We feel like we are looking at the world through perimenopause-colored glasses, and they sure aren't rose colored! It's more like wearing 3-D glasses after you leave the movie theater. Everything is just a bit skewed and it's hard to keep your balance.

This change in how we think seems to be another key aspect of the strangeness of this period of life. Who knows, or cares, whether it is due to age or hormones. It's real. It's difficult. And yet, maybe it is kind of nice to actually pay some attention to how we are feeling instead of worrying about everyone else. Maybe it's okay to focus more on ourselves than others so that we can cover our mental lapses and figure things out when our minds feel foggy. Could it be possible that this is actually Mother Nature's strange way of helping us make this transition to the middle of our lives?

Regardless of your kids' ages, your relationship status, or the stage you're in with your career, this tends to be a time for introspection. You might like dwelling on it or fight its intrusion into your busy day, but we bet this sense of awareness of yourself pops up at least a little.

We think this renewed awareness of "self" truly is a signal that it's a time to focus on you – the real you. That doesn't mean that you actually know who the "real you" is. It means that now is a good time to start thinking about it. Be aware of what is and isn't working. Be willing to acknowledge the things that frustrate you and those that make you happy. For some, the goal is fairly clear, even if the path to get there is bumpy. For others, the easiest way to start figuring out what you want is to identify what you don't want. Once the negatives are identified, the positives can become easier to see.

Unfortunately, for some women going through this evaluation process in the midst of hot flashes, dry vaginas, and love-handles that seem to grow overnight, the soul searching aspect becomes the one area where they can actually take some control. But decisions made in the heat of multiple hot flash moments, such as divorcing a husband who seems emotionally unreachable and irritating beyond belief, may be something you live to regret when your body and your mind calm down. Be very careful not to react too strongly to things now, while you aren't exactly thinking straight.

It seems odd that on one hand we are telling you that you should really think about yourself and what you want and need, but on the other hand we are telling you that you shouldn't really trust what your hormone-addled brain is telling you right now. Yep, here is yet another strange anomaly of this period of life. We have no explanation. We admit it.

We know this is already a self-help book, and we don't want to become a self-therapy book, so we won't continue farther down this path. Just know that if you feel that your brain has gone haywire both in terms of how you are processing things intellectually and in how you're experiencing things emotionally, that is very normal. We encourage you to work with what's going through your head rather than fighting it. While we do advocate being honest with yourself about what is feeding your soul, we also suggest that you try to be very thoughtful and cautious about the major decisions you make at this time of your life. Hopefully, knowing what to expect and being honest with yourself about the mental challenges of perimenopause will be helpful.

Chapter 6

Is There a Hole In My Head? – Your Perimenopausal Mind

Dear Mother Nature: Is this your idea of a joke? If so, you have one warped sense of humor. How many notebooks, sticky notes, smart phones, and whiteboards can one person need??? I spend more time preventing and/or covering up silly mistakes than getting things done. I hate this feeling of mistrust of my own faculties. How am I supposed to continue to appear to be a confident, competent, capable woman when I am feeling anything but? Please, give me my old brain back! If you do, I promise not to call you all those bad names anymore.

The medical community tends to approach changes in brain power as an anecdotal and possibly psychosomatic symptom of perimenopause. Many doctors totally discount or attribute it to aging in general, but we have yet to find a perimenopausal woman who doesn't feel that fluctuations in hormones result in fluctuations in mental functions.

Happily, women who have survived the ordeal and gotten all the way through menopause report that they feel like they "came out of the fog" and stabilized emotionally. That is good enough for us. We are counting on the fact that this will get better eventually. We hope there will be some real quality time in between menopause and dementia!

Remembering to Remember: Memory Problems

There are so many different aspects of memory that can be compromised during this stage of our lives. Sure, all of us struggle at some point, even before perimenopause, to remember someone's name or an important date. Now, however, you may find that it happens with alarming regularity or that you sometimes can't remember the most basic things. And, it may not just be remembering specific pieces of information, like dates or places, although that can happen, too. It can be memory problems that seem like sheer stupidity. You may not remember how to do basic steps in everyday activities, find that you can't remember how to

87

go somewhere you've been going for years, or suddenly realize, in the middle of doing something, that you have no idea what to do next. It can be downright embarrassing! We hope in the future we just won't remember how bad our memory is now.

♀ It doesn't matter to me whether I am a total space cadet because of my hormones (or lack thereof) or the lack of sleep, or whether both are connected. All I know is that there are times when I absolutely cannot focus on what I am doing, can't calculate a tip in my head, and have to look at something over and over again to remember or process it.

♀ I was so relieved to hear that forgetting things is common during perimenopause because I was starting to think that I was getting early Alzheimer's. I know people talk about memory loss and Alzheimer's in a joking way, but I was truly afraid that was what was happening to me. I am so glad I found out that it is typical for women my age. It feels terrible to not to be able to rely on my own brain. I am learning to write everything down.

♀ I don't forget anything. I forget everything!

♀ I frequently lose words, simple words. They just seem gone from my brain, making it difficult to even keep up the appearance of a semi-intelligent woman.

♀ I have left my purse in restaurants multiple times, left it in the shopping cart at the grocery store several times, and walked out the door without it other times. I have never done any of those things except in the last few months.

♀ My most recent perimenopause moment was when I was driving to a good friend's house to play Mah Jongg. I couldn't remember where she lived even though I have been there many, many times. Another great one was when I was at home talking on the phone. I was in a heated conversation, but needed to get to an appointment. So, what did I do? I got into my car and started to drive off. One thing though – I was on my cordless home phone, not my cell phone.

♀ My perimenopausal friends and I have taken to covering for each others' forgetfulness. We know to remind each other before going somewhere to meet to make sure the other person will show up.

When one friend bought tickets online for a play, she forwarded the tickets to me so I could print them out, too. We figured one of us would remember the date of the show and remember to bring the tickets!

♀ If I can remember to get around to it, I am going to invest in the company that makes the little sticky notes. I can't get through a day and remember to do anything without having them all over my computer, the dash of my car, and my bathroom mirror.

♀ Sometimes you just have to laugh at yourself. Other times when it's not so funny, you have to try to keep from crying, like when you can't remember the direction of something in your own neighborhood. What will I be like when I am 60 or 70?

♀ How many times a day can I get up from my desk at work, walk deliberately out into the office, and immediately forget what I got up for?

♀ I could have sworn I had just gotten a refill of my narcotic pain reliever. A bottle of 100 pills, if I remembered correctly, which, of course, was questionable. I spent 2 days looking all over my house, thinking that maybe I had hidden it since I have teenagers in the house. I had the old bottle with a few pills left, sitting right where I always put it in my medicine cabinet. The new one was nowhere to be found. Maybe I had just thought about picking it up from the pharmacy, but didn't actually do it. Nope, the pharmacy Web site clearly stated that I had picked up the prescription a few weeks earlier. After a few very worried days, when I was sure I was going to have to talk to my kids about whether they or any of their friends might have taken it (which I highly doubted), I opened my medicine cabinet to look for something else. Right at eye level, with the label facing right at me, was the brand new bottle of medicine. It had been there all along! It was a slightly different bottle than I was used to getting, though, so even though I was looking right at it, over and over again, I just didn't see it. I felt like a total idiot. I am not sure that I should even be trusted with narcotics at this point!

♀ I was just at a bridal shower where we played a memory game. Everyone had to look at about 15 items attached to an apron that the 40-something-year-old bride-to-be was wearing, then wait a while and write down as many items as you could remember. The person who remembered the most, won. The whole room cracked up when I said, "This isn't a bridal shower game. This is a test to see what stage of menopause we are in!" Sure enough, the winner was one of the kids!

2+2 = ?: Processing Problems

The ability to effectively process information relies on the ability to be aware of the information and to remember it long enough to deal with it. When you can't remember shit, you can't figure anything out, either. Get used to having a blank look on your face!

♀ I feel like I am turning into a man. I used to be able to watch TV, listen to my son talk to me, and think about something else all at the same time. Last night, I was watching TV when my husband started talking to me. Not only couldn't I focus on both at the same time, but I couldn't even process one at a time. I had to ask my husband to repeat what he said. Then, I backed up the TV (thank goodness for DVR at this time in my life!) to watch what I missed. A minute later, I realized I was still thinking about what my husband had said and missed it again. I backed it up yet again and tried to watch. No such luck. It was like the sound on the TV was off. I was staring at it, but nothing was registering. I actually wasn't hearing it because I was still thinking about something else. God, I hope this goes away, although it does give me a better sense of what men go through when they can only focus on one thing at a time.

♀ I had heard that women tend to get forgetful when they are going through perimenopause. What I hadn't heard that totally surprised me is that it isn't just forgetfulness, it is also a total inability to think straight. I feel like I can't process new information or problem solve at all. I can look at a list of things over and over and not see what I am looking for. I can go into my pantry to get something and not see that it is right in front of me. I can read something and not retain a word of it. This is way more than forgetting things or having word retrieval problems.

♀ The feeling of living in a cloud, unable to fully tune into the environment around me, is a big surprise. I had no idea this would happen.

♀ Feeling like I have lost control of my brain is terrifying. If anything gets me to go on hormones, this will be it. I want to feel like I am "me" again.

♀ I used to be the one who could look at the check and almost instantly figure out how to divide it so everyone in the group knew what to pay. Now, I feel like it takes me a few minutes to figure out how much to leave as a tip even when the bill doesn't need to be split. I just can't keep the numbers in my head long enough to calculate anything.

♀ It keeps shocking me that "Sunday," "tomorrow," and "the 15th" are all the same day. Depending on how somebody describes a date for an event completely changes how I think about it. I keep finding that I book multiple conflicting things on the same day without realizing it.

♀ I feel like I did when I had a newborn: sleep deprived, able to only focus on one thing at a time, and lacking any sense of time.

♀ As I drove away from the gas pump, I saw a guy pointing and laughing at me. "What did I do, now," I thought. I looked around inside the car. Nothing seemed wrong or funny with me, so I started checking my mirrors. Nothing in the rear-view mirror. Then I looked at my side mirror. There, hanging from the side of my car, was the entire gas hose. I had forgotten to take it out, driven off with it in my gas tank, and pulled it completely away from the gas pump. I didn't think it was so funny. Thank God it didn't explode or catch fire. I have been filling my car with gas for 30 years. How could I do that?

♀ Yesterday I pulled into the gas station and chose a pump where it would be easy for me to pull out in the direction I wanted to go after filling up. I put my credit card in, then turned around to open the gas tank. I had a moment of panic when it wasn't there. Then I realized that I hadn't given a thought to which side of the car the gas tank was on. How dumb! I had to cancel the transaction, get back in the car, and pull up to a pump that was on the right side. I just hope everyone watching thought I was driving a car I wasn't used to. Of course, I have been driving that car for 6 years.

♀ Lately people are honking at me and giving me the finger while I am driving, but I have no idea why.

♀ Today I pulled up to a stoplight and for some unknown reason put my car into Park. Not 15 minutes later, I put my turn signal on after a stop sign, even though I was going straight. I am not sure that I should be allowed to drive right now.

♀ There I was, sitting and waiting for the light to change so I could go. Then, I realized that I was at a stop sign. I'd like to say this has only happened once, but it keeps happening. You'd think that once I was aware of doing something stupid, I wouldn't do it again, but no!

♀ As usual, I pulled into the garage, stopped just before hitting the garbage cans, grabbed my purse, and started to step out of the car. Then I realized the car was rolling forward. I had forgotten to put it into Park and take the key out. How do you do that? Not even a beginning driver would do that! Thanks goodness I just rolled forward a little and hit the trashcans instead of the house! I was thinking about what I needed to do when I got in the house and just wasn't paying attention. I know now I need to really focus on driving when I am in the car, even if I am just in the garage.

♀ Now I know why people lose their glasses when they are on top of their heads. You sometimes just lose the ability to think logically about the situation. I hope this is only temporary.

♀ I was talking on the phone at work the other day. I all of a sudden could not find my cell phone. I knew I had set it on my desk in front of me. I am opening drawers, looking in my coat pockets and really starting to panic. Suddenly it occurred to me that I was on my cell phone!

Who's Minding the Store?: Perimenopause at Work

It is bad enough to find yourself at the grocery store without a clue what you came in for or to have to fake your way through a conversation with your husband or child when you don't remember at all what they are talking about. These experiences are annoying, but when you are faced with uncontrollable fits of what seems like sheer stupidity at work, it gets very unnerving. The inability to think straight, remember, and behave in an appropriate way can truly feel like a detriment to your work life. Therefore, it is very important to acknowledge to yourself (and possibly to some understanding others) what is going on and find some coping mechanisms to compensate as much as possible.

♀ Twice this week I caught myself walking to the restroom at work undoing my pants along the way! Can you imagine if my boss would have been in the hall? What is with me?

♀ I have taken to carrying a notebook around with me everywhere I go. I write absolutely everything down. I even note when I have done something or e-mailed someone. It sometimes seems like it is a waste of time, but then there will be an instance when I can't remember whether I did something or just thought of doing it. Assuming my eyes can focus and I can pay attention long enough to find what I am looking for, I can review my notes to see what I did.

♀ It seems like I can think of a million things that need to be on my daily to do list while I am in the shower or on my way to work. The minute I am at my desk, the thoughts seem to fly from my head. My solution is to keep a tape recorder and sticky notes in my car so I can record my thoughts at stop lights. Usually I can remember them that long, at least. I wish I could take sticky notes into the shower.

♀ I constantly send e-mail reminders to myself on my phone. Half of my e-mails are reminders to and from myself.

♀ I used to be able to make my to-do list for the day in my head while I was driving to work. Not anymore! I call my own voicemail to leave messages for myself when I am driving.

♀ Thank goodness for the calendar in my e-mail system. I put everything on it. I can't trust myself to remember anything.

♀ My e-mail calendar gives pop-up reminders just before a meeting or appointment is set to start. Of course, that only works when I remember to put all my appointments in the calendar.

♀ I didn't used to carry my phone around with me at work. Now I carry it all the time. I can see my e-mails, send myself e-mails when I am in meetings so I remember to follow up on my commitments, and see reminders about my schedule. It is my electronic brain!

♀ I can't tell you how many times I send an e-mail, then remember something else I should have said, so I have to send another one. Sometimes people get e-mail after e-mail from me as I expand my thoughts, rephrase what I already said, remember to attach the attachment, or answer my own question that I asked in a previous e-mail but didn't really think about until after I hit "send." It is downright embarrassing!

♀ I can focus really well on my work. While I find myself writing down more notes than I used to, I feel like I am doing pretty well on the job. Unfortunately, everything else in my life seems to be falling apart. I am putting so much of my energy into staying focused at work that I am forgetting other appointments, mixing up my days, thinking I have done something at home when I haven't, and just generally messing up.

♀ I have taken to bringing some of my personal to-do's to work and doing some of my work at home. I find that I do better if I can shift from one thing to another rather than trying to stay focused on one thing for hours and hours.

♀ I have started to get work done at night when I can't fall asleep or wake up early in the morning and can't get back to sleep. It works well since I feel that I am not as productive during the day because I am tired and lack focus. Since I can't sleep anyway, it feels good to be productive.

♀ On a morning when I was already running late, the gate at the entrance to the parking garage at my office wouldn't work. I kept pushing and pushing the button as the other cars lined up behind me. Then I realized that I was pushing my home garage door button instead of flashing my parking pass in front of the sensor. God, I felt stupid. I have been parking in that garage for over a year. I hope none of my co-workers saw me with my hand up on my garage door opener!

♀ Everyone at my office knows that I cannot be relied upon right now to remember the schedule. I don't know why, I can remember a lot of other things, but I frequently forget meetings or where meetings will be. Oh, they also know that in the event I do make it to a meeting, I need to make a pit stop in the bathroom before I can go in and right after I come out.

♀ I seem to have lost the ability to remember names. Not a good thing when you're dealing with lots of different vendors, clients, and co-workers. I can remember other things, but not names. I just don't get it.

♀ Even when I carefully write myself a note, it doesn't help if I forget to look at it. Or, worse, if I look at it and in the split second between seeing the note and getting started with whatever it was that I was supposed to do, I remember something else I was supposed to do and get started on that instead. I am getting everything done eventually, but I feel so disorganized when I used to pride myself on my organizational skills. Absolutely nothing has changed other than my hormones, so that must be the cause.

♀ After apologizing numerous times to the president of an organization with which I am affiliated because I kept forgetting meetings and things I should be doing, I decided to explain that I am not normally so absent-minded. I confessed to being in the early stages of perimenopause and that I seem to have totally lost my ability to schedule things at the right time or remember what I planned to do. With a huge laugh she said, "I call that CRS disease – Can't Remember Shit disease. I totally get it!" I can't tell you how relieved I was. She promised that she would, as much as her own CRS disease would allow, try to send me e-mail reminders to help me stay on track.

Mooooood River, Wider Than a Mile: Mood Swings

Angry, joyful, disappointed, loved, optimistic, surprised, afraid, pissed, disgusted, jealous, depressed, elated, stressed, anxious, affectionate, irritated, content, exasperated, nervous, lonely, worried, empty, hopeful, annoyed … phew! And that is just in the last 5 minutes. During perimenopause, we begin to resemble our teen-aged daughters when it comes to moodiness. The difference is that we are experienced enough to know that the emotions we are feeling may not be based on reality. Still, it is very difficult to find that logical place when emotions are running so high (and low and side to side).

♀ How is it possible to feel absolutely furious, but know that you aren't really absolutely furious? I feel like there is a total disconnect between my mood and my mind. I can look at a situation and tell myself I shouldn't be so upset, yet I am.

♀ I am on a mission to appear cool, calm, and collected even though I don't feel that way. There are so many times when I stop myself and count to 10 before talking to my kids because I am so worried that things will come out wrong.

♀ I feel like that little girl in the *Madeline* books. When I am mad, I am horrid!

♀ Out of the clear, blue sky, I sometimes just feel sad and teary. Nothing has changed. There's no reason to feel this way. I just can't control it.

♀ So, I started using hormone cream. Within days I started breaking out in zits, something that hasn't happened for decades. However, my vaginal dryness improved slightly, and I just felt better in a strange, inexplicable way. "What should I do?" I wondered to myself for about a week. Do I focus on how I feel and not worry at all how I look? I felt so conflicted and just so sorry for myself. I mentioned my dilemma to my girlfriend, who had a hysterectomy and has been on hormones for years. She asked if I was feeling teary and sad, too. It hadn't even occurred to me that my mental state could be as affected by my physical state. Duh. It makes sense since we are talking about hormones here. The zits and tears won out. I stopped using that product. Back to trying to find other options for dealing with vaginal dryness and feeling like my period is coming but never getting it. As frustrated as I am with trying to figure out what to do, I am really glad that I opened up to a friend about it. Her one statement helped me put things together and realize that I need to be more careful about side effects, look at the big picture when I try something new, and, most of all, talk to friends rather than keeping my worries to myself! Now, after just a few days off the cream, I feel much less emotional. The zits are even a bit better. Guess I made the right choice. Now I just need to go to the store and pick up more vaginal moisturizer!

♀ I don't feel moody all the time, but my God, there are times when I feel like I am swinging from the highest highs to the lowest lows for almost no reason.

♀ Every so often, for several weeks at a time, I just feel really depressed. Sometimes there are things that justify feeling down, but I feel way more upset than is warranted by the situation. I just can't control it.

♀ I feel old and ugly and clueless as to what to do about it. There are days of emotional lows and some days of feeling good. But, just when I think I may be snapping out of this dark place, it rears its ugly head again. I want something that makes me happy and keeps me happy.

♀ I am bored, depressed, overwhelmed, lonely, and always on the verge of tears. The worst part is that I don't know why!

♀ Here's my advice for women who are going into perimenopause. Advice #1: Hook up with a support group or just a group of friends. For quite some time I secretly feared I had some terminal illness (i.e., AIDS, Ebola, Hepatitis C). I was terrified to get diagnosed with a terrible disease, hence I would stay away from the doctor's office. I thought if I didn't go to the doctor, then I wouldn't get diagnosed with a disease. Some logic, huh? My sister, the nurse, tells me I am perimenopausal and to suck it up. Advice #2: Don't be a girl. I am pissed off that men do not have to deal with this crap. They get to have a mid-life crisis and blow money, party, drink, and date women 25 years younger. We get to hide in our beds all day, wildly depressed, wondering what is wrong with us and why our lives are in the shitter.

♀ My doctor suggested putting me on antidepressants to manage my mood during perimenopause. I am seriously considering it. I think I will be able to cope with everything else much better if I don't feel so depressed.

♀ I wouldn't say I am depressed. I just feel this weird sense of sadness or uneasiness that can't be explained. Once in a while it just goes away, and I feel like myself again. I am hopeful that if I keep learning about ways to take better care of myself, have a good attitude toward my changing body, accept that I can't control my hormones, and try hard not to react negatively even when I feel negative, I can get through it.

♀ The stupidest things are irritating me these days. I am not normally so picky, but I just have no tolerance anymore. It is driving me (and everyone around me) crazy.

♀ Perimenopause has been 5 years of bitchiness. I find that I yell at the people I love the most, even though I know that there is really no reason to be so upset.

♀ I was trying to have a serious conversation with my husband about the various problems caused by perimenopause. We were discussing hot flashes, then I moved on to mood swings and how I get angry even when I don't need to be. That really caught his attention. He perked right up and said, "That's great! Now, nothing is my fault!" This was not the reaction I was hoping for. Now he blames everything on my hormones. I can't be legitimately upset about something. I must be hormonal because I couldn't possibly be right about something!

♀ This is like PMS on steroids.

♀ Having my teenagers assert their independence in order to break away from the parents and leave home is not coordinating well with my menopausal mood swings. Well, I take that back. Maybe it is. Maybe it is just as well that they are driving me crazy and I am driving them crazy. When they go off to college, we might all be relieved!

♀ Having my own mood swings and a teen-aged daughter with hormonal mood swings is not a good combination. I feel bad for my husband and son having to be around such unpredictable females.

♀ The mother of the family projects an energy that sets the tone for the whole house. You know that old saying about how, "if mama ain't happy, ain't nobody happy." Well, I can sense that the whole family's mood is dependent on mine. I may not be able to control how moody I feel, but I am trying really hard not to let it show. It definitely creates a bit more stress on me, but I desperately don't want my family to bear the brunt of my hormonal mess.

♀ I've been feeling down so much that I made a conscious decision to try to control my moods. I am not so successful about getting the negative thoughts and bad moods to go away, but I do seem to be able to add some positive thoughts into the mix. Sometimes I have to work hard to think of things that make me happy and appreciative, but I need that feeling to offset all the negative thoughts that keep going through my head.

♀ I have good days; I have bad days. Life is very unsatisfying lately, but I've managed to put life on cruise control, force myself to have an optimistic attitude, and do nothing life-altering without sleeping on it first!

♀ I am trying to stop and smell the roses, so to speak. When the day has been rotten, I try to find something enjoyable, even if it is a few minutes with a glass of wine and a stupid TV show. I find that I am still moody, but having some good "me time," physical relaxation, and positive thoughts (or no thoughts at all if I can manage it) makes my mood swings less intense overall.

♀ Going to really funny movies with a girlfriend is better than a therapy session. It always has been, but when I'm busy, stressed, moody, and exhausted, going out with the girls seems to be the thing that falls off the schedule. I need to remember that this recharges my battery and makes me feel so much better, even if I laugh so hard I get damp panties!

What to Try: To Cope When Feeling Like You're Losing Your Mind

✓ Stash notepads everywhere so you can write things down. Notes that can stick to the mirror in your bathroom, your computer screen, the fridge, or the dash of your car can be especially helpful if you can remember to move them from the place where you write them to the place where you need to remember to do them.

✓ Make sure to cross off the to-do items that you finish or throw away notes about things that you've already done. Otherwise, it is really easy to overlook the notes regarding what still needs to be done.

✓ Keep a little digital recorder with you so you can leave yourself messages when you can't write things down. Another option is to call and leave yourself a voice message.

✓ Multi-tasking may be more than you can handle right now. Try to focus on only one thing at a time so that one thing gets your full attention.

✓ Talk openly about what's going on with the people around you so they will be understanding and supportive.

✓ Invest in unlimited e-mail and texting on your cell phone so you can keep track of more information in it, rather than in your head.

✓ Learn and use all the helpful features on your phone and e-mail system. There are many that can serve as sort of an external or back-up hard drive for your brain!

✓ Think about thinking. Try to focus more on what you are doing and eliminate other thoughts as much as possible.

✓ Consistency can really help you remember the basics. For example, try to park in the same area each time you go to work or visit the mall or grocery store. Use the same purse and put it on top of your coat or between your feet at a restaurant so you feel it when you get up to leave.

✓ Do not do anything else but drive when you are driving. Don't talk on the phone, text, check e-mails, or try to think about everything you need to do. Focus just on properly operating your car and driving safely!

✓ Try telling yourself you need to remember something, then tell yourself what to remember. The repetition can help.

✓ Say out loud what you need to remember.

✓ Create backup systems. When you schedule something, put it in a hard-copy calendar as well as on your computer.

✓ Use alarms. Program your phone or clock to make a noise just before it is time to do something.

✓ If you can't stay focused on what you're doing, switch to something else for a while, if you can. Just make sure that you find a way to remind yourself to go back to what you were doing in the first place.

✓ Keep the following tips in mind when you are using e-mail or texting:

  • Take a long breath or two before hitting "Send."

- Make sure you attached the right document, completed your thought, and worded things properly.
- Make sure you didn't click on "reply all" unless you really meant to. You don't want to learn this the hard way!
- Don't put any addresses in the "To" section until you have completed the e-mail to prevent sending something before it is complete.
- Check to make sure you clicked on the right names in the "To" box. This is especially important when you are in a rush or when your email system auto-fills names as you type.

✓ Taking your time and double-checking yourself will reduce your stress overall and minimize the extra time it takes to fix things. Doing it right the first time, even if it takes a little bit longer, also helps hide foggy thinking!

✓ When you are feeling irrationally angry or sad, talk to yourself. Remind yourself that you feel that way, but aren't really that way.

✓ When you feel that you are being moody or grumpy for no particular reason, check your body language. If your shoulders are tense and up by your ears, try to let them relax and go down. Same thing goes for your jaw. Relax and try to smile rather than clench. Sometimes, if you let go of the tension in your body, your mind will follow.

✓ Talk to your doctor. If you are having serious mood problems, medications may be an option, even for a short time, to help you through it.

Chapter 7

Who Am I? Who, Who ... Who, Who? – Your Perimenopausal Soul

Are you there Mother Nature? It's me, um ... Geez! Wait, I'll get it! Let's see, I think I am ... no, that isn't right. I'm not that anymore. I know. I'll ask my man who I am. Hmmm, on second thought, maybe that's not such a great idea these days — not so sure I want to know what he might be thinking. I know, I'll look in the mirror. She doesn't look familiar. Actually, she looks just like my mother!

I think I know what I am supposed to be, but that doesn't seem comfortable or familiar lately. I feel like I am asking myself all the same questions, but all the usual answers aren't right anymore.

Whether it is the stage of life you're in, the upcoming or recently passed major birthday, and/or fluctuating hormones, it is very common for women to experience a mental shift during this period. We change from the care-giving, external focus of the previous adult years to a more internal, care-taking mode in the middle years. It is common to feel that you have suddenly lost a sense of yourself and/or that what you always wanted before isn't exactly what you want now. You also may feel frustrated with yourself and others as well as lost and confused. It can be surprising and disconcerting, especially as you are trying to adjust to the changes in your mind and body as well.

Somewhere in Time: Questions, Hopes, Fears, and Frustrations

There are so many unexpected and almost unexplainable changes going on at such a fast pace during this time of your life. It can leave you feeling like you don't know the "right" questions to ask, things to worry about, and improvements to hope for. Don't beat yourself up if you can't help but wonder – as Carrie on *Sex and the City* would say – what this crazy period of life is all about. Just like the columns on that show, sometimes we can just ask the questions, admit our worries, and try to stay optimistic, even when there aren't any real answers.

♀ When I finally figured out that the strange symptoms I was experiencing were probably perimenopause, I did what I always do. I looked for resources to help me understand what was going on in my body and what my options were for dealing with them, so I could make educated choices. I was appalled at what I found. The books showed women who were clearly much older than I was. The "helpful resources" included AARP. One book even listed an association called Help for Incontinent People. That put me off so much that I could barely keep reading.

♀ Overall, this experience of perimenopause is somewhat like being pregnant. Your body changes in unexpected and unpredictable ways. Things that you used to like to eat suddenly don't seem as appetizing. What used to be normal activities, like exercise and sex, don't exactly work like they used to. And, on top of all the physical changes, your mental state seems to change, too. I wish we could count on it getting better in months instead of years.

♀ I don't like being so focused on how my body is declining. I wonder if, at some point, you just become used to it and stop thinking about it so much.

♀ If I could go even a few months with symptoms that are fairly predictable, I could cope with this so much better. I would find natural methods to control them, feel some sense of control, and adjust to whatever the problems are. But from month to month, and sometimes week to week, everything changes.

♀ Purging my closets, files, and basement is my new pastime when I am sleepy but can't sleep. I love going through things that haven't been used or looked at in ages. Organizing and consolidating makes me feel like I have accomplished something. Who needs that old, pressed corsage from prom? Why the hell did I ever save so much crap from high school? My kids certainly aren't ever going to care about seeing them. I can't even remember what most of those things are, even though I know they used to mean a lot to me. I feel so virtuous for cleaning up and being organized. Best of all, it takes minimal brain power. In a strange sort of way, it also makes me feel good to see what used to be important to me compared to what is important to me now and makes me feel better about where I am in life.

♀ How do I figure out what is really bothering me? There are a million things that sit inside of me and just stew. I find myself questioning my life: why am I here, what am I supposed to be doing, what does my life mean, and what does anything mean! I can't quiet my brain. Do other people think this much about things?

♀ I am trying really hard to remain involved and engaged. But, I have major parental burnout! I don't even remember my 30's as I was so involved being in the PTA, a Girl Scout leader, room-mom, team mom, etc. I am coming down the home stretch here, but running out of steam. I feel distant and apathetic. I have no energy. This is so not like me and leaves me feeling very guilty about not knowing how to make things better.

♀ I have had it with being the caregiver. I am mother, wife, and daughter, and I don't want to do it anymore. I feel guilty about it but the feeling doesn't go away. I feel like my whole life is about taking care of everyone else's needs. Don't I get to have needs?

♀ I have an overwhelming urge to run away on a daily basis. I won't of course ... my family needs me. I love my family and I have always considered myself happy with my life. I don't know why I feel so unsettled all of the sudden.

♀ One night I stood outside my house looking through the windows at my family, my home, my "life." I felt like a complete stranger looking in on someone else's life. In some ways, it looked so familiar and in others, it seemed like I did not even belong there. Why is the familiar suddenly so unfamiliar to me?

♀ I look at myself and think that maybe I am not the person that I have always thought I was. I have had this image of myself all my life that I was a certain way and had certain characteristics, but suddenly I find myself wondering if maybe I am not any of those things after all. I feel like a stranger to myself, if that makes any sense.

♀ At least during pregnancy, there were lots of books that told me what to expect and when to expect it. How are you supposed to prepare yourself when perimenopause can take anywhere from 3-10 or more years and when there is no real information on how/what women experience, and much of what I am experiencing is considered anecdotal and "unproven" medically?

♀ I've heard that women tend to take after their mothers and grandmothers with respect to their menopause experiences, but all the older women on both sides of my family had hysterectomies for one reason or another. I wish I could talk to them about what they went through with perimenopause.

♀ I'll just have to be the one in my group of friends who opens her mouth first and speaks about the unspeakable. I just hope some of them can relate to what I am going through.

The Chicken or the Egg: Is it Age or Hormones?

It's important to recognize that one of the challenges of perimenopause is recognizing and dealing with the signals that indicate we are moving into a very different stage of life. Other than not having periods anymore, it can be hard to view the outcome of this transition in a positive light, like we can with puberty or pregnancy, though. We will just be older and, we hope, wiser!

♀ I never gave this time of life a thought. It always seemed so far away. I expected it in my late 50's or 60's, not in my 40's, so I feel unprepared for it.

♀ The most surprising aspect of perimenopause for me is just the fact that I am old enough to be at this stage in my life.

♀ I am so tired of hearing my doctors start every comment with the phrase, "women your age."

♀ My sister-in-law was just diagnosed with breast cancer and is about to have a double mastectomy. I always knew that someday this would happen to someone close to me. Some day has come. It makes me feel old and vulnerable.

♀ I certainly hope that everything I go through now with perimenopause isn't going to be repeated again when I am older and post-menopausal. Once is more than enough.

♀ I am terrified that this is a preview of old age. I don't feel old chronologically, but I have a lot of the symptoms that I think older people experience. I definitely do not want to feel this way for the rest of my life.

♀ Wrinkles, saggy skin on my neck, getting far-sighted, gaining weight around the middle, having thinning hair on my head, incontinence, and getting forgetful. Is this menopause or just old age? My husband is almost 20 years older than I am and going through some of the same things.

♀ When I complained to my gynecologist during my annual exam that I am getting forgetful and having trouble seeing, he said those are just things that everyone has to deal with as they get older. He wasn't willing to discuss how they might be related to perimenopause. I'm only 42, though, so aging doesn't seem like it should be the only issue here!

♀ I can tell that I'm in a different stage of life because actors my age are now being cast in the mother roles.

♀ An alarming number of products in my medicine cabinet have the words "age-defying," "firming," or "anti-wrinkle" on them. It seems like I went from worrying about zits like a teenager to worrying about sagging and wrinkles like an old woman virtually overnight.

♀ There are so many more steps in my morning and bed-time routines now. I use multiple lotions, take lots of vitamins and herbal supplements, and actually floss once in a while. It seems like these extra steps are helping me look and feel younger, so I am going to keep doing them.

♀ I don't know or care whether it is that I am old enough to know what I want or hormonal enough not to care about pissing someone off when I say what I want, but I am way more assertive now than I have ever been before. I just don't have the time or energy to waste trying to explain, coddle, or cajole. I am much more direct and to the point. I don't think everyone around me likes it, but that is just too damn bad.

♀ How in this day and age of information, could I, a well-educated, professional woman who prides herself on being well read, not have known about perimenopause? I am absolutely shocked to find out that so many symptoms occur before true menopause. I totally thought that your periods stop and then you start feeling miserable as you adjust. I thought I had years to go before I even had to think about starting to learn about this. Now suddenly and unexpectedly I am in the middle of it when I am just barely 50. I feel cheated out of years of my life. Just when I thought things would be calm and settled, I am in total upheaval emotionally and physically and am not enjoying this time when my kids are off at college and my husband and I are both stable in our jobs. And, I feel sorry for him, too. I don't think he is able to enjoy it as much either, because of my moods. What's worse, when I finally get through this, it will probably be his turn for a midlife crisis. I guess I should be looking forward to our late 60's at this point because I don't see a light at the end of the tunnel until then!

♀ I am 49 years old and have been married to a man that I love for 12 years. My problem is that I feel everything in my life is going horribly wrong. I hate my body and the way it is changing. I must be going through "the change" because I just feel so emotional. I look at 20-something year-olds with envy and jealousy. The worst part is that I have never been and will never be unfaithful to my husband, but for the first time in my life, I'm actually craving the excitement and newness of a different, younger man. I plan on working through this and staying married for many years, but is everything supposed to be upside down like this? Is this a "midlife crisis?"

♀ What are we supposed to be changing into? It sure as hell isn't into a butterfly. A moth, maybe! During puberty we were changing into a woman. When we were pregnant we were changing into mothers. Now it feels like we are changing into old women. I feel like fighting against that kicking and screaming!

♀ During the first years of perimenopause, I felt like I was turning into someone completely different. I wasn't so sure I liked her. Now that I am almost through this stage, I find many things about myself that I really like. There are even some things that I wish had changed earlier.

♀ I think this is a fabulous age and I love this phase of life. I've always been interested in health and wellness personally and professionally, and I believe that is one of the reasons I feel so great at this time. I notice that I don't recover as fast from either a night of too much food, or too little sleep, or too much wine, and that is okay. Sometimes you go for it and just enjoy the moments without worrying. That, too, is a gift of being older. If I don't feel 100%, I don't let it affect me as much as I may have been inclined to at a younger age.

What do You Want to be When You Grow Up?: Exploring Options for a Different Stage of Life

Your moods change by the minute. You feel like you don't know what is going to happen to you tomorrow. There are things you can't remember from yesterday. No wonder it seems hard to get a really good sense of where you've been and where you are going these days. While this tends to be an introspective time for women, that doesn't necessarily mean that you will be able to be reflective in a highly productive and organized way right now. In the past, you knew what stage would come next. In the first half of our lives, we knew that we would go through the various stages of school, probably marry and have children, and perhaps build a career. Now, the choices aren't so clear. Our preferences aren't, either.

It's hard to know what we want when the options are so new to us and this stage of life isn't something that we dreamed about as girls or planned for as young women. However, that doesn't mean that you can't pay attention to what means something to you these days. Weigh the pros and cons of the various options that have presented themselves to try to decide what direction to go in next. And, because of the freedoms this stage of life can offer, such as reduced childcare responsibilities and/or more career choices, remember that what you choose today doesn't have to be what you stick with for the rest of your life. Focus on what feels right now and aims you in what feels like a good direction. Then later, if things change, whether they are external factors or your own internal thoughts, you can readjust for the new reality.

♀ What I want at this age has turned out so differently from what I thought I would want. I am certainly not raring to go full steam ahead career-wise now that my kids are out of the house. Really, I just want a nap. The things that used to interest me don't so much anymore. I feel like I am in search of who is going to be the new me.

♀ Decrease of ambition. A growing lack of interest. Detachment. Depression. Oh, joy. Just what I need at the point in my career when I should be able to seriously focus on career growth after years of putting myself in the backseat to my kids' needs.

♀ For the past 6 months I have been so depressed and lazy. I work from home but do just enough to get by. I am so dissatisfied with my life and am looking for something, but I have no idea what it is.

♀ I just want to leave everything, and I have everything! I have a loving, devoted husband, 3 awesome kids, a beautiful house, and a successful business. And still I'm not happy! It is not a good feeling to wake up each day, not like where you are, and just want to leave. To be painfully honest, I don't want to be a wife and mother anymore. It is so upsetting to feel this way. I am totally spent, lost, and just don't want to think anymore.

♀ I started having all of these unsettling feelings and emotions in my mid-40's. I did not understand them at the time and, unfortunately, I tore my life apart and ripped my marriage to shreds before I figured it all out. I have tried to explain to my husband that it was nothing he did and something was wrong with me, but, I don't think we will ever be able to get back to where we were.

♀ I was sure that when my kids were in high school or college, I would be ready to hit the workforce full steam ahead. I worked part-time in the past and planned to go full-time at this point. Unfortunately, I am exhausted now. I want to curl up with a good book far more than I want to work full time. It's sort of embarrassing to admit this. Plus, I worry that if I don't ever really focus on my career and do everything that I held back on doing before, I will regret it at some point. I wish I was as excited and ready as I thought I would be.

♀ Is it really that Madison Avenue has realized that women our age and stage of life are a huge target market so they are running tons of ads for bladder control products and medications, support bras, and other age-appropriate items, or is it that I am suddenly paying more attention to them? When I was pregnant it seemed like I saw pregnant women everywhere I went. I actually got frustrated that so much of my focus was on one aspect of my life. I feel the same way now. I just need to get out from underneath this perimenopausal haze and focus on the rest of my life.

♀ I am in search of a new hobby for the large amounts of spare time I have now that my kids are older and gone most of the time. I used to crave unrestricted amounts of time to read or work in the garden. Now I have more time for that than I want. I want something that captures my attention. I want something that makes me feel excited and happy even when I am moody and down. I want to feel young and active again, even when I am swamped with work and family obligations. Nothing seems to fit my needs right now.

♀ I read a million books on pregnancy when I was pregnant. My favorite was *What to Expect When You're Expecting*. I loved how it just gave me a sense that what I was going through was normal and to be expected. I also loved being able to read ahead in the book and find out what was going to happen next. That is what I want now – a sense that I am not alone and will get through it and feel better on the other side. I also want to know what to expect about my life after I am done with menopause.

♀ My grandmother really did think that having kids was her primary purpose in life and that she was somehow less important once she could no longer do that. My mother was one of the first Baby Boomers. By the time she was going through menopause, her biggest issue was how it would affect her at work. Even though her generation started to talk about it, they didn't have much information. Her perspective is that hormones are the answer to everything. Neither of them can really share the kind of information I crave about how to get through this and what my options are for the next stage of life. I am going to have to stick with my girlfriends to talk me through this!

♀ I am getting close to actual menopause, but now my husband is showing signs of his own little man-o-pause. He seems moody and his sexual functions seem to be a bit different. I think he also feels a little out of whack with who he is and what he wants. He was very supportive of me, so I guess it is my turn now. I am glad this waited until I am through the majority of the difficult time of perimenopause. I don't think I could have dealt with that while I was trying to deal with my own issues.

♀ I have seen so many couples get divorced just after their kids go off to college. I used to think that they had waited until the kids left or that the husband was having a midlife crisis. Now I know that perimenopause or menopause probably contributes to the trend, too. I have seen women go completely ballistic. I have had my own times when I was so totally irritated that I wanted to just divorce my whole life and start over, but I kept telling myself that I was feeling that way for no reason other than hormones. If it doesn't go away soon, I will start exploring my options for hormones or herbal therapies, but I am going to fight really hard not to let my phantom feelings affect my marriage.

♀ It is strange to be at this stage of life without being clear about what I want. My thoughts, moods, and preferences seem to be changing so much that I can't get a clear picture of where I am going. I am just trying to stay away from the things that I really don't want, be aware of the things that seem to interest me a little bit more, and make a gradual shift rather than some huge, dramatic change that is just a reaction to everything going on right now. This applies to my work, my relationships and all my activities.

♀ I thought that if I worked hard and made good choices during my 20's and 30's, I would be well on the path to having made great achievements. While I have accomplished a lot, I don't feel like I am on the path that will take me into my future. I am no longer even sure that a "path" exists – whether it is because of the wisdom I now have due to my age or from the state of the world. I just wish I didn't still have so many choices to make about my life and career. I had really hoped to be more settled, if nothing else. I am tired of trying to figure out where to go and what to do next. In some ways, I wish I was older and past this stage.

♀ Every time I go several months without a period, I hope that this is "it," the real thing so they won't come back. Then I'll get a period and feel like I am starting all over again. I am so tired of this waiting and wondering what will come next. I just want to be formally through with perimenopause already so I can focus on other things and not have to try so hard to compensate for how I feel physically and mentally.

♀ The first few years of perimenopause were hellish. I truly felt like I didn't know who I was or have any control over my life. Now, I still have the symptoms, but I also feel like I have a bit more perspective. This is just another transitional period in my very happy life. I recognize that I am not really depressed, I just sometimes feel that way and need to try my best to help myself get out of it when it happens. I have great girlfriends who commiserate with me, so I don't feel alone. I even am starting to feel like I could get to like this new me who is interested in different things, able to focus on life from a different perspective, and at a stage where it is okay to be a little bit more self-centered.

♀ It certainly is strange to think I will be 50 next year and, at the same time, it is exciting and fabulous. The way I see it, we have 2 choices about getting older: either embrace it wholly and roll with it, accepting it all, good and bad, or fight and deny it. I don't like the latter approach; it's too draining.

♀ I asked my 95 year-old grandma how menopause was for her. She said that she went though it "early," which was in her early 40's. (We haven't come very far in 50 years in our understanding of what "early" menopause is!) She said that when she got all "wound up," my grandfather would pack her in the car in the middle of the night and just drive her around until she calmed down. It really made me feel good to know there was some family precedent for what I am experiencing and that they were able to figure out something that helped. It was strange how much it helped me to think of my grandmother feeling that way during perimenopause, but getting over it. She clearly recovered her composure, and she surely recovered her cognitive skills. She remembers more than I do these days. And, she worked hard and got far in her middle-aged years. If she can get through it and thrive, I can, too!

♀ When I was younger, it was important to make career choices that would point me in the right direction so I got where I "should" be. Now, the timeline is so much shorter. By definition, unless I want to keep working forever, I need to be pretty close to where I "should" be. I find myself surprised that I can make shorter-term career decisions because I don't need to try to figure out where I want to be in 20 years. I only need to think about where I want to be in 5 or 10 years. After that, I am going to cut back on work and travel more with my husband.

♀ Yes, the physical uncertainly of this stage of life is challenging. I feel like I don't know myself. On the other hand, I kind of like the idea that my body is my own again, even if it misbehaves. My time is my own again now that my kids are independent. My husband and I are reconnecting in new ways and going back to some of the things we did before we had kids. I am kind of glad I am going through perimenopause now because it is forcing me to be introspective and really think about how I want to be as I move into the next stage of life.

♀ The fluctuations in the economy mirror the fluctuations in my moods. It's so not fair that just when career and finances should be starting to get easier, they're essentially out of my control. When exactly do I get to relax and enjoy? I'm not saying I know what I want, but I do know that I would be so much better at handling economic stress if I wasn't also dealing with my own personal issues at the same time.

♀ Suddenly, our family choices about work and income are so different. We aren't as worried about saving up for college because the kids are already there. We are in the house we always dreamed about. I feel like my choices can be based more on what I want and like than on their financial ramifications. It feels really good, although I have to admit that I am so used to focusing on how much I could earn, that it is a bit strange. I can get used to it, though!

♀ I am leaving the "should haves" and "could haves" behind. I am also trying hard to leave guilt behind. I am old enough, experienced enough, and strong enough to make sound choices about what I want to do next, even if they don't seem completely logical to others. It feels really good to do things for me, rather than for what others will think of me.

What to Try: To Feel Like Yourself Again

✓ Talk to your girlfriends. This time of life is like being pregnant or a new mom. It is so important to have a group of people who are navigating the same course as you, at the same time as you. Even if they don't have any answers, it will feel good to talk.

✓ Talk to your partner. The more he understands what is going on with you emotionally, the more supportive he can be (theoretically speaking, anyway).

✓ Talk to a therapist. Sometimes, it takes a professional to sort through everything. Since this can be a very introspective, philosophical time of life, it might help to talk to someone totally objective.

✓ Talk with women who are older than you are, both so you can feel young and so you can learn about what life is like at their stage of life. It might be better than you think!

✓ Read a variety of books, fiction and non-fiction, to help you feel like you aren't the only one going through this.

✓ Try various options to manage your physical symptoms. When your body feels better, your soul might very well feel better, too.

✓ Try something new for relaxation, such as yoga or meditation.

✓ If you've always dreamed of writing a book, learning to knit, traveling to a far-off place, redecorating your house, or going back to school, for example, this might be a great time to do it. If not, maybe it is a good time to explore how to do it, start to prepare to do it, or at least think more realistically about doing it.

✓ If you can't dredge up the time or energy to do a new hobby or activity now, it still might be helpful to think about it and get ready now. Then when you reach that post-menopausal "zest" that we have heard about, you'll be ready to go for it!

✓ Our attitudes and expectations about menopause and aging can affect our sense of self and even our ability to cope with physical changes as we transition. If you let yourself think that there will be something to be ashamed of, that you are no longer truly a woman,

115

that you are somehow less valuable when you can no longer produce children, then the transition to menopause can be very upsetting. Instead, try to look forward to not having to deal with periods. Celebrate this new stage of life when your family is less dependent on you. Use diet, exercise, or treatments that make you feel better. Most of all, laugh over the outrageous experiences you face these days. You can't choose whether or not to go through this stage, but at least to some degree, you can control your feelings about going through it.

○ ○ ○

SECTION V

SEX SYMBOLS

So far, we've been talking about changes that are going on within you, your body, mind, and soul. Although it's probably been fun to focus on just yourself, it's time to address the world around you. Lord knows, the way you feel physically and mentally affects how you interact with others. You aren't going through perimenopause while the rest of your world is paused. Life goes on around you despite how you feel or how you react to things, so being the good girlfriends that we are, we need to talk about that, too. And, since we are really good friends, we are going to focus on two of the most important aspects: sex and the person with whom you have sex.

We recently received one of those chain emails that contained the following pertinent information (the author apparently wanted to stay anonymous):

> A university study conducted by the Department of Psychiatry has revealed that the kind of face a woman finds attractive on a man can differ depending on where she is in her menstrual cycle. For example: if she is ovulating, she is attracted to men with rugged and masculine features. However, if she is menstruating or menopausal, she tends to be more attracted to a man with duct tape over his mouth and a spear lodged in his chest while he is on fire. No further studies are expected.

We think that sums things up nicely. Clearly, we are at the point in our lives when both our bras and our partners need to be more supportive. If you've been in a long-term relationship when you enter perimenopause, your partner may start to wonder what alien has invaded his partner. If you are in a newer relationship, you may not feel totally comfortable sharing your deepest, darkest bizarre experiences with that special someone. After all, those difficult physical and mental challenges that we addressed in the first part of the book are hard to talk about with almost anyone, not to mention someone who is really important to you, who might not be able to relate to your struggles, or who might be going through some of his own transitions at the same time.

No matter how hard it is, though, we encourage you to find a way to create a new "normal" with your partner. This strange period could last years and years. It isn't like PMS that is something to suffer through for a few days on a fairly regular schedule. If you don't let him know, he might think that something else is going on. Of course, there might be other things going on in your relationship, too, but those will be even harder to deal with when you are hot, uncomfortable, hormonal, and exhausted.

In most cases, our partners can be more supportive if we let them into our world a little bit. Maybe you won't be able to explain the whole situation to him, but he might be able to understand key pieces. Maybe you don't feel comfortable talking about it, but you can hand him this book and ask him to read it. Or, maybe you can get together with other couples and you and your girlfriends can talk to each other about perimenopause in front of the guys, so they can hear it, but you aren't talking directly at them. Find a way. Take the risk. Make things better for yourself, for him, and for your relationship.

Note: This section is also relevant if you have a female partner who hasn't reached this stage of life yet. Just please forgive the many references to "he" or "him." If you are in a relationship with another woman who is going through perimenopause at the same time you are, we wish you all the best and encourage you to read through this book together!

Chapter 8

Too Hot to Trot – Your Perimenopausal Sex Life

Dear M.N.: I wish I could tell you, "Not tonight, honey," instead of telling my husband! I really want to want sex, but I just don't. I find it seriously twisted of you to take away my sex drive at almost the exact time my husband expects me to be entering my "peak." It is cruel and unusual punishment.

For years, it was hard to have sex because the kids were always around, I was exhausted from caring for them, or it was the wrong time of the month. Now that I have fewer periods and we have more time, sex should be better, not worse! Instead, I am dry, hate my body, and am hardly ever in the mood.

Making love is like making a delicious cake (a triple chocolate one, with chocolate chips, chocolate mousse filling, chocolate frosting, and chocolate sprinkles, just for example!). There are many ingredients that go into the cake. But, unless all the ingredients are good quality, all are put into the batter, all are in the right proportions, and the oven temperature is just right, the cake can end up tasting anywhere from bad to inedible!

Here are just some of the ingredients typically involved for a woman to get in the mood to "make a cake:"

- comfort and security in her relationship
- ability to turn her brain off
- attractive feelings about her partner
- emotional connection to her partner, and
- at least a fairly decent body image that day (or a dark room)

Don't forget, we will also need:

- 2 cups of energy
- 1 cup of time
- a dash of privacy

- a day when we have shaved our legs
- a time when we don't have our period, are about to have our period, or have just ended our period
- oh, and our favorite show can't be on TV

Now we need to pray that our partner doesn't do or say something stupid to screw up this very precarious balance, like:

- coming into the bedroom and passing gas just as he is about to get in bed, or
- oozing the odor of the bratwurst with raw onions and sauerkraut he ate for lunch, or
- looking at you, raising his eyebrows, pointing to his middle-aged version of an erection, and saying, "Oh yeah, you know you want some of this!"

Yes, it is a delicate recipe, but we are experienced bakers! At least we were before Mother Frickin' Nature started sucking the estrogen out of our batter. That bitch. And who wants cake made by a sweaty, crabby chef with whiskers and fifteen newly found extra pounds of flesh?

Our partners, who typically could be counted on as "a sure thing" are starting to change, too. Men also go through some substantial physical and emotional changes as they age. Testosterone levels can change, which can cause symptoms very similar to perimenopausal symptoms in women (hot flashes, night sweats, fatigue, mood swings, irritability, and depression). These changes also have sexual effects. Many men experience decreased libido (of course it is not the men who are with women with lowered libidos – that would be too easy). They also can experience difficulty getting or sustaining an erection and/or difficulty reaching orgasm. These changes can pack a huge emotional wallop. Being a man, he may then retreat, seem disinterested in sex, feel the need to prove that he can still be a sexual, virile man, or anything in between.

Let's look at the picture that we've painted: on one hand, we have a woman who is feeling lost in a body that seems only to vaguely resemble the one she knows as her own. Now, put her with a partner who is either having his own aging issues or isn't yet and doesn't get what has happened to this woman he feels like he knows so well. How does a cake ever come out right?

What's in it for Me?: Your Sex Drive

We know that when our batter is messed up in any way, it is hard for us to bake. We aren't like men, who seem to be able to use sex to feel better almost no matter what the problem is and sometimes actually use sex to solve their problems or make themselves feel better. Women, on the other hand, need most things to be pretty okay beforehand. When we feel like we've lost our minds, our body is doing strange and unusual things that leave us feeling far less than sexy, and we have a strange sense of not being ourselves, it can be difficult to get cookin'!

♀ How am I supposed to feel sexy or "in the mood" when my vagina is bone dry, I have gained 20 pounds in the last year, I am constipated, and my pubic hair is taking over the world? I don't want my husband to think it is because of him, but getting naked is truly the last thing I feel like doing.

♀ I used to have a pretty healthy sexual appetite. Over the last year it has just disappeared. Most of the time I have to pretend to be in the mood. I used to feel so proud about the great sex life I had with my husband.

♀ My husband's friends told him that women lose their sex drives when they go through menopause. Now he is petrified that I won't be interested in sex anymore since I am in perimenopause. Any time I am not in the mood, I sense him thinking that this is the beginning of the end. I feel this pressure to ease his fears and my own fears about the possibility that it could happen. What if I do totally lose my sex drive? How will it affect our relationship?

♀ You know how they say that women hit their sexual peaks during their 40's? I was really looking forward to it. Unfortunately, I think I blinked at the wrong time. Who knew my peak would last for about a split second?

♀ I think menopause is perfectly named. It describes exactly how I feel. I want to put "men-on-pause!" I have absolutely no interest.

♀ Back when life was crazy with the kids and we hardly ever felt like we had the time for sex, I really wanted it. Now I have all the time I ever wanted, but between the vaginal dryness, the yeast infections, the weight gain, and my general bitchiness, I hardly ever want sex anymore. No, I take that back, it's not even that I don't want sex. I literally can't stand the idea of it. I feel myself sort of cringing sometimes when I can tell my husband wants to make love. I feel horrible about it, but I don't know how to change how I feel.

♀ I want to want sex, but I just don't. What do I do? Do I pretend to be interested for my husband? I feel so bad because I don't want him to feel undesirable or unattractive, but I literally have zero interest.

♀ My sex drive became non-existent. I did a no-no and borrowed some testosterone cream that my girlfriend had gotten prescribed by her doctor. She was getting testosterone shots, so she no longer needed it. I figured I could give it a try and, if I liked it, go get my own prescription. At first, it did very little, so I upped how much I used. I kept upping it until I felt my sex drive come back. Then, I realized that I had upped it too much. Sex was all I thought about. I needed it, and was miserable if I didn't get it. It gave me a whole new perspective on men. Now I understand why they are so focused on sex and some like porn and hookers. It is a physical need, not an emotional choice. Once I backed off and used less, I felt what I thought was a normal sex drive. I think lots of women could benefit from using testosterone, especially if they talk to their doctors about it and use it the right way.

♀ Over-the-counter progesterone cream made an almost immediate difference to both my vaginal dryness and my libido. I actually caught myself thinking about sex in the middle of the day. That hasn't happened for ages! Of course, it has other effects that I didn't really like, so I need to figure out whether or not I will stay on it.

♀ I know a lot of people say that their drive goes down, but mine is actually better. No little kids anymore, more sleep, much more comfortable in my relationship, it's all good. My hubby is pretty darn happy about it too. We both hope it stays that way!

♀ For some unknown reason, I find that I am more in the mood for sex during my rare menstrual periods than at any other time. My hormones must be different at that time, or maybe just feeling moist instead of dry helps.

♀ I am finding that more than ever, if my mind is not there, my body ain't goin' either. If I am distracted thinking about everyday life stuff, worries, or stresses, it is almost impossible to get in the mood.

♀ My sexual desire seems to fluctuate with my hormones. I can get totally horny in the middle of the day, but have no drive at all at night. I can also have several nights in a row when I badly want sex, then have months with no desire at all.

♀ Although my sex drive is much lower, sex is actually more satisfying now than it used to be (as long as I use lubrication).

The Lube Tube: The Physical Aspects of Sex During Perimenopause

As with practically everything else during perimenopause, sex may take a bit more physical effort and preparation. Happily, if you can get in the mood, there are things you can do to help sex be more comfortable and enjoyable. If you want to keep the cake-baking analogy going, you can think of it as needing to preheat the oven and grease the pan! (Want to bet that the next time you have sex, you think about baking a cake? Maybe it will help.)

♀ I feel so uncomfortable with the changes that are happening with my body. It is not like me to feel so insecure, but I have no idea how my husband could even be remotely attracted to me right now. He is trying so hard to make me feel desirable and beautiful, and I want to believe him. But, then I look in the mirror and I have no idea what he sees. I hardly recognize my own body.

♀ I know that women are supposed to enjoy going slow and taking time with sex, but when I am so dry, going for a long time, even with lubricant, can be more painful than pleasurable. I know it is taking him longer these days, and I should be accepting of that, but there comes a time when enough is enough. At that point, I can't pretend to want to keep going. I always feel bad for him afterwards, but I don't want to be rubbed raw.

♀ Sometimes, sex just feels like irritating friction. When it goes on and on, it feels like he is trying to start a fire without a match!

♀ I have times when I will bleed a bit after sex, especially if I didn't use lubricant.

♀ Even when I am in the mood and get a bit of natural lubrication, it just isn't like it used to be. It is more watery feeling instead of slippery.

♀ I keep reading about vaginal dryness during perimenopause, but I am experiencing exactly the opposite. I am getting wetter than ever. When it first started, I was afraid I was leaking urine. Thank goodness my husband likes it.

♀ My guy and I were fooling around and let some warming massage lotion get where it shouldn't. It felt like I was having a bonfire inside my vagina! Lesson learned the hard way: do not use something that isn't intended to be vaginal lubricant as vaginal lubricant.

♀ Is it because I am less sensitive down there that I hardly feel him inside me anymore, especially if I use lubricant? Or it might be that my husband isn't quite as firm and large as he used to be? Both?

♀ I tried generic lubricant, and I don't recommend it. It turns into the stuff left on a piece of paper after you use an eraser. Yuck!

♀ Try olive oil. It works. Really!

♀ I am so grateful that my doctor suggested vaginal hormone cream. Not only do I stay lubricated enough for sex to be pleasurable, but he says it will help prevent vaginal atrophy.

♀ When I first started to need lubrication, I felt defective. Plus, it seemed like I was back in my college days when I had to get up, go to the bathroom, and insert my diaphragm. It was a pain and got in the way of the mood. Things got much better when I finally admitted that this was going to stay part of our sexual routine. I moved the tube of lube into the drawer by my bed. Best of all, instead of putting it on myself, which I hate doing, I either put it on my husband or I give it to him to put on me. Treating it like massage lotion makes it fun rather than functional.

♀ It takes me a lot longer to get in the mood and a different type of foreplay than I used to like. My husband teases me that the "right spot" is a moving target. Luckily, he looks at it as a challenge to find it.

♀ I was in the middle of having sex with my partner the other night and I literally tooted right in his face! Totally involuntary loss of control of those muscles! I was so humiliated. What is happening to me? I was eventually able to laugh about it with him but at the time I was mortified.

♀ My partner and I were getting ready for bed and it had been a playful, flirtatious evening, so it was pretty clear that there was going to be some lovin' that night. I went to the bathroom and when I got up to flush, I noticed quite a bit of blood in the water. "Shit!" I yelled from the bathroom. I put in a tampon and got in bed with one disappointed guy. After 24 hours of putting in tampons and pulling them out clean, I realized that the blood was not coming from my vagina, but instead from my rectum! I went to the doctor the next day for my very first rectal exam. Doesn't get much better than that! Not one ounce of dignity left now. Anyway, I have an internal hemorrhoid, an anal fissure, and an appointment for a colonoscopy. Age, constipation, and babies – the culprits, according to my doctor. Yeah baby, I am sure my man can't wait to make passionate love to a constipated old lady with hemorrhoids and butt fissures.

♀ Don't stop worrying about getting pregnant just yet, ladies. I was 47 and had tubal problems when I got pregnant! The doctor was even shocked.

♀ I love looking forward to the time when I won't have to worry about getting pregnant or deal with birth control. At least there will be one really great outcome from this experience!

It Takes 2 to Tango: Your Sexual Relationship

Sometimes you can't have your cake and eat it, too. You can't expect your partner to be responsive to your needs and feelings unless you do the same for him. Although your appetites might be different now, you have to find a way to make it work for both of you.

♀ My husband is trying so hard. He wants me to enjoy making love. He wants me to feel fulfilled physically and emotionally. He wants this aspect of our relationship to be strong, as do I. He would do anything I asked him to do. I wish I knew what to ask him.

127

♀ The touches that used to feel so good haven't just stopped feeling good, they now feel downright irritating. My husband must be so confused. This feels like the beginning of the end of our intimate life together. I really hope I am wrong and that I will feel normal again soon.

♀ My husband used to get upset if he thought I was faking an orgasm. These days ... not so much! Now, he is more concerned about whether or not I am faking being asleep when he's in the mood!

♀ I want to make our sex life better, but I feel so apathetic about it. My husband says that I only use sex to patch things up temporarily when he is upset with me about it. He could be right. I wish I wanted it more and for different reasons.

♀ For a couple of years, it was my body that wasn't reacting as it should during sex. I was dry, dry, dry. Now, it's my husband's turn. Although he can get started okay, he can't always finish. I hope we get back in sync at some point soon!

♀ If I am going to be totally honest here, the changes in my husband are really killing it for me. He doesn't get really hard anymore and it seems to take him forever to finish. How do I ask him to talk to his doctor about taking something to help?

♀ I also seem to be ultra-sensitive to smells, sounds, and touch these days. It is like everything is intensified and not in a good way. Something that has been so familiar to us for so many years now all of the sudden feels strange. I think we both spend a lot of time worrying and thinking about it because it's seriously affecting our sex life.

♀ Sometimes, our sex feels like the monkeys in the cage at the zoo. The male monkey is humping away on the other monkey, never once asking her how her day was or what she wants or needs.

♀ How do I go about telling my husband that I really don't feel like having sex most of the time? His sexy/provocative talk is driving me nuts. The less I want it, the harder he tries. I used to love how much he was attracted to me. Now, I want to scream at him to please just give me room to breathe.

♀ I know that if he's not getting his needs met, he will at the very least start to build up and harbor resentment. What if my disinterest is the beginning of the end?

♀ It is so ironic to see all these commercials for things that help men get bigger more frequent erections so they can enjoy sex more. All those men that are getting more into sex have wives or partners who probably want sex less and less!

♀ I find it helps if I tell my guy how often I realistically feel like having sex, and then make sure that I follow through. If the frequency is pretty regular, he seems much happier and less resentful.

♀ This notion about how a man will stray if his needs aren't met is blackmailing bullshit on the one hand, but scary close to the truth on the other. Although we all have to forgo gratification at some time or another, I am really scared that my lack of interest (which I can't control) leaves him vulnerable to other women.

♀ I want a close, intimate relationship, but sex isn't such a big thing for me now. I am single, in my late 40's, and worried that no man is going to want me when he can have a younger, sexier, more sensual woman instead. After all, my ex left me for someone 15 years younger.

♀ How do you coordinate a male midlife crisis with perimenopause? It is not a good combination. I am bitchy as hell. He is desperate to look and feel young. I have little interest in sex; he is out to prove what a man he still is. I truly worry about him leaving me for a younger woman. Sometimes, I wouldn't blame him. I would leave me for a younger version of me, too.

♀ I never so much as looked at another man then, out of the blue, it happened to me. I had an irresistible urge to "reconnect" with an old flame online. I have always been loyal and completely in love with my husband. Now, I can't stop thinking about and wondering about how happy I really am. My husband can sense that something is "off," and I don't know how to explain any of this without hurting his feelings or scaring him. I used to think women like this had flawed characters and just plain made bad choices. Now, I am not sure about anything. I don't recognize myself. I am sort of afraid my virtual connection might become something real if I am not very, very careful. I am sure that I already crossed a line just by contacting him.

♀ I wonder if our relationships affect how we feel about sex. When women are in long-term relationships, like 20 years, many seem to be fine with feeling less sexual now. On the other hand, my friends who are divorced and in exciting new relationships seem very into it!

♀ I hardly have any desire for sex, but I definitely want my husband (who still very much wants it several times a week) to be happy. So, while I will occasionally make it clear that I am not in the mood, and he is respectful of that most of the time, I do sometimes just kind of let him go for it. Sometimes I will end up getting in the mood and finding that I enjoy it. Other times, I just want him to take care of himself. It makes me happy that he is happy, even if I am not having a great sexual experience for me. It also makes me really pleased that he still finds me attractive and sexy. It just takes looking at sex a little differently when I am not really in the mood.

♀ Just knowing that my husband wants to touch me and make love to me is enough. I don't have to have the same kind of urge that I used to.

♀ My guy is ignoring my dryness and difficulty reaching orgasm. I am ignoring his spare tire and difficulty reaching orgasm. Such is life. At least we are still having sex and trying to make each other happy.

♀ I hate to admit it, but I do sometimes have sex with my husband just enough to keep him happy. It's less than romantic in some ways, but also loving in others. I want him to be satisfied even if I'm not.

♀ This is the morning after starting vaginal estrogen cream. My husband had been in the mood last night, but there was just no way I was going to let anything else in there, so I turned him down. This morning we had a really good talk about what is going on with me. I asked him to please just give me a little time, without the resentful attitude that sometimes crops up when he feels it is too long since we've had sex, to figure out this vaginal dryness problem. I promised him that I did want him, but sex is not something to look forward to when it actually hurts. I reminded him that I wasn't just ignoring the problem since I had called the doctor and gotten a prescription that I hoped would improve things. I assured him that it was physical and had nothing to do with him. He surprised me and just cuddled and talked with me for a while. It was very reassuring and supportive. It was a very nice way to start the day.

♀ For me, good sex requires good emotional intimacy. Right now, I don't know how to find that in myself or in my husband. Should I fake it? I don't want to hurt his feelings. I feel like my husband is testing me to see if I am pretending to be in the mood or faking an orgasm. He knows I am having trouble with the early stages of menopause and knows that loss of sex drive can be a problem. He doesn't seem to care about most of the other symptoms, but he definitely cares about this.

♀ When we were first together, my partner and I had our own little language for sex. Over the years, as sex got more routine, it pretty much went away. Now that we have to discuss sex again, since it isn't working so well for either us, those code words make it so much easier to talk about what is going on and what we can do to help each other.

♀ In a strange sort of way, it is kind of nice to focus on sex again. In some ways, having to figure out what works for my dryness and lack of interest and his limpness is a good thing. After years of taking sex for granted, like it was a step in getting ready to go to sleep, it is now something that we both want and pay attention to. We are really aware of each other and our needs, just like we were in the beginning when we were getting to know each other.

♀ On a dark, icy night with temperatures of less than zero, I called my husband on my way home from work. The kids had finals, I was exhausted, and there was no way I was going to cook, but the kids wouldn't want to go out. I suggested that I pick up prepared food to eat at home. My husband, without my asking, offered to do it instead. Not only did he pick up dinner, but he picked up a few other grocery items that he knew we needed. That was the biggest turn on I had felt in a while! It just made me feel relaxed, supported, and cared for. Instead of coming home stressed, I came home grateful and happy. Needless to say, we had a nice time in bed, too! If he hadn't been so helpful, there is no way in the world that I would have been in the mood for sex that night. I told him so, too!

What to Try: To Enhance Your Sex Life

✓ If what used to work to get you in the mood doesn't work anymore, try different things. Maybe you need to find a different kind of foreplay.

✓ Don't forget birth control just because you haven't had a period in a long time. You might still be able to get pregnant.

✓ Talk to your doctor about vaginal hormone cream to increase your natural lubrication and avoid vaginal atrophy. That alone might improve your sex drive.

✓ Talk to your doctor about other prescription hormone creams. (There are various options.)

✓ Carefully try over-the-counter hormone-type creams and lotions, such as progesterone cream. Be careful to follow directions and tell your medical professional what you are using.

✓ Invest in lubricant. If one type doesn't work well for you, try another one.

✓ If, after a while, intercourse becomes physically uncomfortable, try taking a break, adding some lubrication, or switching to another type of sexual pleasure. Make sure your partner knows that it isn't that you don't want the sex, it's just that intercourse is making you physically uncomfortable.

✓ Turn the process of getting lubed up into part of your foreplay.

✓ Plan a get-away. When you aren't dealing with your every-day life, it might be easier to get in the mood.

✓ If your sex drives become incompatible, discuss a "schedule" or days during the week that you will have sex. It doesn't sound spontaneous, but the partner with the higher sex-drive benefits because he/she knows that his/her needs will be met and not put off until "later." The lower-drive partner can relax knowing that sex will happen and when, which may alleviate the pressure and the "dance" of uncertainty every night.

✓ Talk to your partner about it being okay to have some times be just for him, some times be for you, and some times being for both of you.

✓ Talk to your partner about his physical issues. Maybe if he can take something to get a better erection, sex will work better for both of you.

✓ Instead of being irritated with your partner for not being able to figure out what is and isn't working for you these days, talk to him about it, move his hand to the right place, initiate what you want, or do whatever it takes to make sex pleasurable for you. He will probably be very, very appreciative, especially if it makes you want to have sex more often.

✓ Try different options when you really aren't in the mood. Sometimes say, "no" and be okay with it, no matter his reaction. Other times, if he is really in the mood try a little foreplay. You just might be surprised and find yourself getting in the mood. If you do, hallelujah! If you don't, maybe you can focus on taking care of your partner. If that doesn't work, maybe he will be pleased that you at least tried. If your partner is desperate, it is okay to "give" him sex in order to make him happy. Even if you aren't doing it for you, it can be a caring, loving thing to do.

✓ Don't assume your partner understands what is going on in your body or how it is affecting your sex drive and your feelings during sex. Explain it to him, explore it with him, make him feel like a part of the solution. Saying it out loud and getting his perspective could end up making things better in many ways, physically and emotionally.

✓ Let your partner know how you feel about your own lack of sex drive or physical changes that are affecting your sex life. Let him know that you wish it was like it used to be and that you are scared it may never be again. That might help him talk about how he feels about the changes in your sex life. Just knowing that you want to want sex might make him feel better, too.

✓ Even though it is hard to understand it sometimes, remind yourself that men express love and giving through sex. He is probably not just trying to satisfy his own needs, although that is certainly a part of it.

He's also showing you that he loves and desires you, regardless of the recent changes in your body, mood, and spirit. That's a good thing!

✓ Use your words. Sometimes the sexiest thing in the world is saying, "I love you," "I would marry you all over again," and "I love my life with you." Remember, the brain is the most important sex organ!

o   o   o

Chapter 9

Looking at the World Through Guy-Colored Glasses – Your Partner's Perspective on Perimenopause

Dear Mother Nature: This is her husband. Leave my wife the fuck alone.

As important as our feelings and needs are, each of us is just half of the equation in a relationship. You have to get outside yourself sometimes, no matter how intense your internal focus is right now, and acknowledge, respect, and respond to your guy. In both the short-term and the long-run, making sure he is okay and that your relationship remains strong will give you what you ultimately want – a partner who is supportive and caring as you go through this stage of life and the ones still to come.

Who Are You and What Have You Done With My Wife?: His Perspective on Your "Change"

Since how your partner feels (physically and emotionally) affects you, we decided to gather some input from some guys who are living through the perimenopausal years with the women they love. Interestingly, we found that guys who are living through this stage secretly wanted to talk about it.

The guys who had an idea about what was going on wanted to find out whether their wives' experiences were normal. They were proud of their knowledge and accepting attitude toward perimenopause and hoped that they could help other men feel more comfortable, too. The guys who didn't know what was going on had a real eye-opening experience when we brought them together with more educated guys and their wives/girlfriends for some very open, very uninhibited conversation.

We are not so sure that any of these guys would be so willing to discuss their own hemorrhoids, sexual dysfunctions, weight gain, hair loss, or emotional issues if they were the subject, but they sure enjoyed sharing their perspectives on our experiences and how it affects them!

♂ I think I I'm the kind of guy who likes to sleep with the window open and the fresh air coming in, but not when it is 20 degrees outside! My wife is hot at night even if it is below freezing.

♂ I've learned not to take it personally when my wife can't stand to have me touch her during the night. She finally explained that it just makes her really hot, but not in the good way.

♂ At least with PMS, I could sort of predict when it was going to happen, see the usual signs, and get out of the way. With her symptoms now, I never know when they will be there, and they aren't the same as they used to be.

♂ It was disorienting when I could no longer predict when my wife's periods would come. A couple of times in the past I even planned our vacation schedule around it. Now, neither of us has any idea. I feel sort of out of sync with her.

♂ My wife acted like she thought I should know exactly what she was talking about when she told me that her hormones were starting to change. I was an idiot and said something about how her hormones change every month and how was this different. I truly didn't know.

♂ I had no idea what to think when my wife told me that she was starting perimenopause. I knew absolutely nothing about it, good or bad. Was I supposed to? If so, how? No one talks about it.

♂ My wife is smack in the middle of "the change" or whatever you call it. She doesn't talk to me as much as she used to. She is always hot (or cold), does not like me to see her naked anymore, is dressing differently, and is spending more time with her girlfriends. She says that she feels "different" and needs space to think. Is this normal? Should I be worried?

♂ My wife looks so different than she used to. I finally got to know her post-baby body, and now it is changing again. I have to remind myself often that my body is changing too. I guess this is a part of what it means to grow old with someone you love.

♂ I am not surprised that my girlfriend is getting moody and has irregular periods and a lower sex-drive. I am surprised that it is happening when she is in her mid-40's. I was expecting it later in life.

♂ If I could just get sex once in a while, I would be a lot more understanding about all the other shit. I find myself looking at other women and wanting them. It makes me angry with myself for feeling that way and angry with her for changing.

♂ I think that since we have commercials for erectile dysfunction on network TV, we ought to be able to talk about what is happening to women, too.

♂ It is not just us guys who are not functioning the way we used to. All the ads for bladder control, weight control, hair creating and hair removing, antidepressants, etc. are for both men and women. It is like the beginning of a total body malfunction once you hit 40.

♂ I can handle all the physical stuff my partner is experiencing. We have always been very open about those things. She doesn't care that my hair is thinner, my neck is saggy, and I have gained weight around my middle, too. I am just really struggling with her mood swings. I have seen so many couples break up at this time in their lives. I would hate for that to happen over hormones. That would feel like we broke up over something that isn't real. I know that hormones are real and making her feel upset in a real way, but there isn't anything real to get upset over. Intellectually, I know she can't control it, but at the time, it seems like she should be able to.

♂ A relationship is a give and take. If she isn't so interested in sex for herself right now, I appreciate that she sometimes is interested just for me. There have been many times when I have taken care of her sexual needs, and now there are more times when she is taking care of mine. There's nothing wrong with that.

♂ When my ex-wife first started going through this, I took it personally when she was less interested in sex and being close physically. I made it even worse because I got irritated. She took that as me being insensitive, which really irritated her. If I had to do it over again, I would be more supportive of her feelings. If I had, I think everything might have been better and easier for both of us.

♂ I can tell that sex just isn't doing it for my wife anymore. She isn't as receptive when I touch her, and sometimes it seems to irritate her more than please her. I wish she would just tell me what I can do differently. I really love her and want to please her, but I am not a mind-reader.

♂ I know that sex isn't terribly important to my wife. I think she looks at sex as a way to show me that she loves me and wants to be with me. That's good, but I wish I could make her want it and love it, too.

♂ The other night my wife told me she thinks of me as more of a best friend than lover and spouse. We have been so close for our entire marriage. I thought women wanted a man who would love them unconditionally. This is affecting our sex life and my mental state.

♂ I'm now divorced from a previously wonderful woman who turned into a raving lunatic after having a total hysterectomy (with ovaries removed) at 41. She refused to admit that she had experienced instant menopause, that her behavior was being affected by the lack of hormones, or that she should consider getting medical treatment or even alternative therapy. She literally went from being the person I had loved for over 10 years to someone I didn't know and didn't want to know. I called her doctors, begged her to get follow up care, and did everything I could think of to be supportive, but she said she wanted a separation. When her response to my leaving a rose in her car when she was at work was to tell the police that I was stalking and harassing her and having a restraining order issued against me so I couldn't even go into my own home, there was nothing more I could do but file for divorce. Even then, I told her I would do anything if she would go to the doctor to manage her hormones. I am absolutely convinced that our marriage is a victim of untreated instant menopause. "Temporary insanity due to hormone fluctuations" should be a category that you can choose when you have to state the reason why you are petitioning the court for divorce!

♂ I'm happy to see my wife getting involved in new activities now that the kids are older and she has more time on her own. I also have to adjust, though, because I am used to her being more focused on our home and our family. Sometimes she thinks I'm upset about it, but it's just that I'm not used to it.

♂ My wife suddenly seems so much more assertive and sure of herself. She is like that everywhere, including the bedroom. I have to get used to her being more demanding and having different needs.

♂ Talking with the guys about the changes our wives are going through at this stage of life isn't going to happen, but I can see a few of my friends getting a wandering eye. I don't think it is because they no longer find their wives attractive, but more that they feel like their wives are sort of ignoring them lately.

♂ One of my teen-aged sons just told the other that he should go find a video to watch on "manstruation" because he was acting too hormonal. I guess hormones have turned into the scapegoat for practically everything around here.

♂ Here is a funny blurb that has floated around the Internet (without any authorship credits – the poor guy is probably too afraid to put his name on it). I pass it along to my friends who have wives or girlfriends going through perimenopause. This handy guide should be as common as a driver's license in the wallet of every husband, boyfriend, male coworker, or significant other.

The Hormone Hostage knows that there are times when all a man has to do is open his mouth and he takes his life into his own hands!

Dangerous: What's for dinner?
Safer: Can I help you with dinner?
Safest: Where would you like to go for dinner?
Ultra Safe: Here, have some wine.

Dangerous: Are you wearing that?
Safer: You sure look good in brown!
Safest: Wow! Look at you!
Ultra Safe: Here, have some wine.

Dangerous: What are you so worked up about?
Safer: Would you like to talk about it?
Safest: Here's my paycheck.
Ultra Safe: Here, have some wine.

Dangerous: Should you be eating that?

Safer: You know, there are a lot of apples left.
Safest: Can I get you a piece of chocolate with that?
Ultra Safe: Here, have some wine.

Dangerous: What did you do all day?
Safer: I hope you didn't overdo it today.
Safest: You go take a bath while I clean up!
Ultra Safe: Here, have some more wine.

♂ I got this email forwarded to me from another guy who is suffering through his wife's hormonal changes. Since PMS is also due to hormone fluctuations, it works for PeriMenopauSe, too. Coincidence? I think not!

Things PMS Stands For: Pass My Shotgun, Psychotic Mood Swing, Perpetual Munching Spree, Puffy Mid-Section, People Make me Sick, Provide Me with Sweets, Pardon My Sobbing, Pimples May Surface, Pass My Sweatpants, Pissy Mood Syndrome, Pack My Stuff, Potential Murder Suspect

♂ I don't take anything my wife says personally. Actually, I consider her a temporarily insane person – a mental patient, if you will – because that's what she seems like sometimes. I'm now in my own midlife crisis, so her changes seem to make more sense now ... well, as much sense as totally illogical behavior can ever make.

♂ Asking for counseling was tough for me. It just didn't feel very manly. But, I eventually discovered that the best way to get the help you need is to ask for it. Things are getting much better.

♂ My advice for men is to remember that you cannot "fix" her, and trying to understand it is almost impossible. It is not about you. It is about her, and she can't help it.

♂ Okay guys, you probably won't believe me now if you are in the middle of this, but I can tell you from personal experience that once she is through all this insanity and change, you are going to love what you see. Hang in there! I did, and my wife has emerged again, only more beautiful, creative, self-assured, wise, peaceful, and yes, sexier than ever!

The Man in the Mirror: His Perspective on His "Change"

There seems to be some uncertainty about the hormonal changes that men go through as they age. Some professionals throw around the controversial term "male menopause" while others may refer to it as "andropause," "viropause," or "andro decline." Testosterone is the hormone responsible for a man's sexual development and drive. Testosterone levels typically begin to decrease between the ages of 40 and 60, but it can begin as young as 30 for some men. There is a big difference between the hormonal changes in men and women as they age, however. It is time, literally. The testosterone decline in men is very gradual, typically lasting decades. Some men will even have normal testosterone levels into old age, which is why much older men can still father children.

Although there are men with low testosterone levels who don't experience symptoms at all, there are some men who report having symptoms similar to those experienced by perimenopausal women, such as hot flashes, mood changes, fatigue, loss of sexual desire, and sleep disturbances. Many men will also experience some form of erectile dysfunction or impotence as they age, including an inability to get an erection, difficulty sustaining an erection, and/or problems reaching orgasm.

In addition, whether it is caused by something hormonal or it is just age related, men sometimes experience the infamous "midlife crisis." With physical and psychological changes going on, this can be (almost) as frustrating a time for a man as it is for a perimenopausal woman. Following is what some guys had to say about it.

♂ I've always had to get up during the night to urinate. But now, instead of getting up once, I am getting up multiple times. I don't fall asleep again as easily as I used to, either.

♂ I guess I thought that prostate exams, colonoscopies, and bifocals were for old men. Either I am old in my late-40's or my expectations were wrong!

♂ It is very typical for me to fall asleep on the couch in the middle of the afternoon, even if I am watching a great football game. I just doze off and can't help it.

♂ Thanks to all the ads on TV about erectile dysfunction, I think I would be comfortable asking for medication if I couldn't get it up. As of last night (I don't take anything for granted), I can still get it up, it just doesn't quite stay up like it used to or get up as high, if you know what I mean. I wonder if there is a medication for erectile *mal*-function. I am scared to try any of those "male enhancement" products.

♂ For me, the midlife crisis is about realizing that I truly am in the middle of my life. There are things that I've always wanted to do that I need to do soon. I don't have time to waste anymore because I already feel like my body is getting older. I want to do what I can as soon as I can.

♂ My wife kept bitching about how I was acting like I was having a midlife crisis and that I should get over myself because I don't have to deal with hormonal changes like she does. I looked it up online and found that some of the "symptoms" of a male midlife crisis are loss of interest in work, health issues related to stress, reminiscing about the good old days, desire to focus on a life goal, depression, lack of interest in the marriage, desire for a fresh start, pessimism, irritability, and increased drinking. I hate to admit she's right, but that does sound like me. Actually, it sounds like her, too. Maybe we are both going through the same type of thing at the same time. Fuck that!

♂ My wife is hardly paying any attention to me. I don't know if she is bored after so many years of marriage, can't stand that I have gained some weight and lost some hair, or is just having a bad reaction to her own changes. I can't help that I need some attention and affection, though. I love my wife and will try to make things work, but I won't put up with this forever.

♂ I love my wife dearly, but I sort of understand how men could feel the need to be with younger women. I am having a hard enough time with the physical and emotional changes I feel. When it is clear that my wife has no interest at all in sex, it is really demoralizing.

♂ I miss the emotional connection my wife and I used to have. She seems not only less interested in sex, but less interested in me. I have to admit that I miss having a woman make me feel like a man.

♂ My wife complains of feeling like she's not herself and wants something, but doesn't know what it is. I feel exactly the same way.

♂ I can't cope without an emotional connection with my wife. We need to talk, interact, and have fun together. I am trying to give her the space she seems to need right now, but she can't keep ignoring me forever, regardless of what she is going through.

♂ Sex is something really important to me, but now the emotional connection is as important, if not more so, than the physical release.

♂ I had a low sex drive when I was in a loveless marriage. Now that I am with a loving and emotionally open woman, my sex drive is back more than ever. I feel like I'm 18 again.

♂ I don't like the changes I am feeling in myself. I'm trying to shake things up by buying nicer clothes and other things that I can finally afford, working out and laying off the donuts, and trying to go to exciting places. It is now or never. What the hell. Maybe I am the cliché of a man in a midlife crisis, but now I know why men do it. It is time they got to have some fun for themselves instead of taking care of everyone else.

♂ I have an urge to make things more exciting and interesting. I hope my wife is game for it.

What to Try: To Help Your Guy Understand What You're Both Going Through

✓ Explain perimenopause to him by using the following analogies as appropriate:

- A hot flash is like taking a big mouthful of horseradish, only you feel the burn all over your chest, back, face, and head, not just in your mouth and nose.

- A hot flash is like wearing multiple layers of 100% wool clothes on the very hottest summer day in the tropics.
- A hot flash is like swallowing a space heater stuck on the highest setting.
- Having episodes when your mind and eyes just won't function is like going to a really important business meeting when you have a horrible sinus infection, and you can't see or think straight.
- Having sex when your vagina is bone-dry is like getting a hand-job with a sandpaper glove.
- Having sex when your vagina is dry is like trying to shove a square peg in a round hole.
- Walking around when your vagina is dry is like having sandpaper in your underpants.
- Having a gushing, unexpected period is like walking around with the seat of your jeans sopping wet.
- Having a gushing unexpected period without having sufficient protection in your panties is like pooping in your pants.
- Having a gushing, unexpected period that overflows the pad is like suddenly vomiting all over yourself or wetting your pants in public.
- Having to run to the bathroom constantly for a woman in perimenopause is what a guy can expect when he gets older and has prostate problems.

✓ Remind him that he may very well experience hot flashes, mood swings, and other lovely side effects, too, as he goes through his own change in testosterone levels.

✓ Be willing to talk to him about what you are experiencing. Although it might be intense to you, he may not have a clue about what is going on with you unless you explain it to him. He is just a man, after all!

✓ If he is having a hard time discussing feelings with you, try starting out by first discussing the technical aspects of what is going on. For example, describing the proven medical facts about how hormones affect weight, mood, vaginal dryness, etc. might help him absorb the information. Maybe he will be able to have a more emotional conversation once he has had the chance to address it first from a more logical perspective. Plus, he really might not know about the effects of hormones and need some education.

✓ Communicate, communicate, communicate! Encourage him to talk about how he is feeling physically and emotionally. He might be going through some transitions, too. Unless he is really in touch with his feelings, he might not really be able to discuss this, but it's good to make sure you find a way to bring this up in a way that can't be taken as a criticism of his sexual prowess or his strength as a man. It's worth a shot if done carefully.

✓ Encourage him to see his doctor if he is experiencing real physical problems. There are treatments for atypically low testosterone levels.

✓ Encourage going to a therapist, either together and/or just him. Therapy and/or medication can help many people. Be open and encouraging.

✓ Learn as much as you both can, understand as much as you can. Knowledge is power, while the unknown is scary and can be very damaging.

✓ Make a pact with each other to find ways to address the changes in your lives in a way that strengthens your relationship.

✓ Remember that he may be feeling very unsure and insecure. Tell him often the things you love about him. Make sure he knows that he is attractive, important, smart, funny, whatever! Don't just assume he knows. It is good for you, too, to remind yourself of the things you love about him.

✓ Make your relationship a top priority. Go on dates, don't let your sex life disappear, and get away together even if you don't feel like it!

✓ Have him read this book! If you want him to be sure to understand specific sections, highlight or put notes in the margins before you give it to him. Or, read it together. Maybe there are things that you are experiencing that would be easier to discuss if he reads about it, rather than if he hears it from you.

○ ○ ○

SECTION VI

THE LIGHT AT THE END OF THE TUNNEL

Congrats. You've made it through the stories of hundreds of women who are in the midst of the bizarre experience of perimenopause. Some may have applied to you; others didn't. We assume you skipped over some, laughed so hard you peed over others, and couldn't wait to talk to your girlfriends about a few particularly strange ones. These years in the middle of our lives really are a strange period, aren't they?

Now it's time to move one step further. Now that we've learned what we can from each other, let's hear from women who have gone through perimenopause and are now post-menopausal. We hope you are pleasantly surprised and start to feel good about what comes next.

Whether you can't wait to get through perimenopause or you dread menopause, we hope that understanding both will ease the transition. Keep acknowledging your experiences, finding the resources you need, and knowing that you are normal and wonderful no matter how hot, hormonal, and hysterical you are right now.

Chapter 10

It Ain't Over 'Till the Menopausal Lady Sings – Life After Perimenopause

Dear Mother Nature: It has been 14 months since my last period. I feel like I have gotten to the light at the end of the tunnel. I still haven't lost the weight I gained in the last few years. I also still have an occasional hot flash, and my skin definitely doesn't look as young and fresh as it used to, but I am comfortable with who I am, physically and mentally, and ready for whatever is next in my life. I feel like I have come out of the fog, and I am comfortable with what I see. In fact, I feel more "present" and more like myself than I have in my whole life.

PS: This was all part of your master plan, wasn't it? Maybe you're not so bad after all.

It can feel like we are frantically pushing the "rewind" and "fast forward" buttons when we are in perimenopause. Our hormones are fluctuating like crazy so we experience most of the symptoms that are traditionally called "menopausal" symptoms. Our bodies and minds are trying to find a specific hormonal level at which to settle so we can create a new sense of normal.

Menopause, the year after our last period, can feel like we are truly on "pause," waiting to see if there will be another period, waiting to see which, if any, symptoms will continue for the long term. Then from what we are told and the studies seem to report, it might feel like the "play" button has been pressed when we truly reach the post-menopausal stage. We will start to feel who the new "me" will be. Our lives will get back in focus.

We feel it is appropriate to show you the light at the end of the tunnel by sharing some of the experiences of post-menopausal women. And, just to be fair, we are including stories from women who experienced significant perimenopausal symptoms, women who took or take hormones and/or used alternative therapies to address their perimenopausal symptoms, and women who had fairly easy transitions. The good news is that no matter what our perimenopausal experiences or choices are, we will likely feel much better about ourselves, our bodies, and our lives when we are post-pause!

This is Your Brain on Menopause: The Mental Effects of Menopause

Many menopausal women report feeling that once they are officially post-menopausal, their minds clear up, they can think again and remember more. Please, God! In addition, after all they've already been through with perimenopause, post-menopausal women also seem to feel a sense of accomplishment and joy at finally getting through such a difficult period.

♀ I didn't realize just how bad my memory was until it started to get better again. I must have looked like an idiot for years on end.

♀ Now that I feel better, I am not spending so much of my mental energy on thinking about how I feel physically and trying to figure out what to do. When I am not spending so much time thinking about how I feel, my brain seems to have some excess capacity to think about other things. I am less forgetful, more able to pay attention to what I'm doing, and just more alert in general.

♀ My mother promised me that I would feel like I had come out of the fog. I had a hard time believing her at the time, but now I know she was right.

♀ I just reached the official point of menopause and am now post-menopausal. It's been 12 months. No more panty-liners. No more birth control pills. No more counting days on my calendar to try to predict when and if my period would come. No more counting months, praying that it wouldn't come again. Hopefully no more hot flashes and dryness. We shall see. Whatever comes, it can't be worse than what I've already been through.

♀ The 3 P's are gone: pregnancy, periods, and PMS. I am in heaven! White pants are even back in my wardrobe! Best of all, I no longer feel like there is a huge part of my brain power being sucked up with trying to figure out what my body is doing hormonally. I just don't have to think about it anymore, which seems to free up a lot of brain power for other, more important things.

♀ I heard about how my daughter talked with her friends about what they were experiencing in the years leading up to menopause. I wish I had been brave enough to talk about it when I was in my 40's instead of thinking I needed to keep it all hidden. Seeing how open she is with her friends has helped me be more open with my friends. There isn't as much to discuss when you are post-menopausal as when you are perimenopausal, but every so often something happens, and it's nice to be able to feel comfortable talking about it. In fact, sometimes I even go to my daughter for advice these days.

Hasta La Vista, Baby: Your Body after Hormones

We are thrilled to finally be able to give you good news: since you are already experiencing most of what you thought were "menopausal" symptoms now, during perimenopause, this is likely going to be the hardest part. Things will get better. Although you will probably still experience some physical symptoms when you are post-menopausal, they will likely be less frequent and less intense than there were during perimenopause.

♀ I am sort of glad that I didn't know what to expect from perimenopause before I got into it. There was no sense dreading something I couldn't control. I was just really surprised when it started when I was so young. I had no idea what to expect. Then, once I was in it, I felt like I was on a trip without a map or navigation system. That was when I wished I knew more. Now that I am post-menopausal, I just wish I knew more about what symptoms I can expect to continue to have and how long they will last.

♀ I have 3 pieces of advice for women who are in perimenopause: get a fan, get a good pair of tweezers, and remember to do Kegel exercises to maintain strength in your pelvic floor. You will be able to evaporate the sweat from your brow, make sure you don't have big long whiskers growing out of your chin, and minimize urinary leakage and vaginal atrophy. What more does a girl need to know? And, most likely, you will continue to need them for many years to come!

♀ I had horrible stress urgency throughout perimenopause. I would frequently leak urine, not just when I laughed or coughed. When I got past menopause, though, it got much better.

♀ Many of my symptoms went away after menopause, but vaginal problems still bothered me. My doctor gave me hormone cream to insert vaginally to minimize the vaginal atrophy and dryness that I was experiencing. It makes me feel much better, plus I really think that it helps me avoid urinary problems. It seems like everything stays in place better when I use the cream.

♀ I went through medical menopause, but it was still menopause. My advice, no matter how you go through menopause, is that if you choose to take hormone replacement, be patient. Trying to find the right dosage is challenging. I started taking 1.0 mg of one hormone, but now I am on 0.025 mg. Finding the right dose takes months and can even change over the years. Don't be afraid to work with your doctor to make adjustments on your dosages.

♀ I was very frustrated when I first went on hormones. I went from fluctuating due to lack of hormones to fluctuating because of the hormones. After about 6 months of adjusting the hormone levels, though, I started to feel much better and much more regular in my moods and my body.

♀ I love my hormones. Even if they find that hormones shave years off your life, I don't care. I would rather be stable, supple and satisfied now.

♀ I'm sure that my breasts didn't just get droopier. They also got heavier. As long as the hot flashes don't come back, though, I can deal with this.

♀ After going well over a year without a period and considering myself completely done with bleeding, I was shocked to see blood in my underpants. It scared the shit out of me. I rushed home and got right onto the Internet. I was reassured when I found that there are lots of normal reasons for post-menopausal bleeding, some of which include hormone imbalance, rapid weight loss (definitely not the cause for my bleeding), and stress (a much more likely cause in my case.) Since the articles also pointed out that uterine cancer can be another reason for bleeding, I did make a doctor appointment. I was very scared to hear what the doctor would say, but much less terrified than I would have been if I hadn't already known that it is relatively common. Thank goodness everything was fine.

♀ When I was in perimenopause, I hated how often I would wake up in the middle of the night, hot and with my adrenaline pumping. I had real trouble falling back to sleep. Now, if I wear flannel pajamas to bed, there is a 50/50 chance that I will wake up naked in the morning. Apparently, I can now wake up long enough to throw my pajamas off, but I don't stay awake long enough to even remember it. I can live with that.

♀ I knew nothing about perimenopause before I started. All I had heard about from menopause was hot flashes. Boy, was I surprised to experience night sweats, hot flashes, weight gain, widening around the waist, hair in new unfortunate places, changes in mood, feeling like I was losing my mind (and my keys, purse, glasses, children, etc.), vaginal dryness, unpredictable and strange periods, decreased sex drive, unusual fatigue, depression, difficulty concentrating, memory loss, painfully slow metabolism, painfully large appetite, restlessness, and uncertainty before I was even 50. Surprise! Happily, most of those things have gone away now that I am officially post-menopausal. The biggest relief was not having any more periods and having the long-lasting bloating go away.

♀ I was recently doing some online research about menopause. I found a list of 35 symptoms related to menopause. I counted up 30 or so that I experienced to some degree during perimenopause. (It was a long 9 years!) Now that I am post-menopausal, there are only a few that continue to bother me, and they are less severe than they used to be.

♀ I used to be able to attribute my personal thermostat issues, heart palpitations, skin eruptions, and weight gain to perimenopause. Now that I am post-menopausal, I am not sure whether or not I can still claim hormone fluctuations as an excuse. I worry and am conscious about my health in a whole new way.

♀ In the early years of being post-menopausal, I still had many of the same symptoms that I had during perimenopause and menopause. Now, about 10 years later, most of them have either gone away or gotten a lot better. So, after about 18 years, I finally feel like my hormones have leveled out. It's about damn time.

What to Expect About Not Being Able to Expect: The Loss of Fertility

The loss of fertility used to be a major physical and emotional aspect of the adjustment to menopause for women in previous generations. These days, unless a woman is experiencing menopause much earlier than average or trying to get pregnant in her 40's, this aspect of menopause doesn't seem to disturb women all that much anymore. Of course, it is a milestone in our lives, so it means something, but the anguish and the sense of not being useful for child-bearing just doesn't seem to be there.

♀ There is not one tiny ounce of regret over losing the ability to get pregnant, but I did get a few moments of sadness when my teen-aged daughter first started getting her period. I realized that we would never have our periods on the same cycle and share that womanly experience.

♀ After so many years of planning for periods, counting months, and using birth control, it is really strange not to have to think about these things at all. I'm sure I can get used to this, though!

♀ I can't imagine how menopausal women must have felt a few generations ago when child-bearing was a woman's primary function. It must have been really difficult for them to lose their purpose in life. I am very glad I was born into this generation.

♀ I don't want another baby. I am perfectly happy that my kids are teenagers now. Nevertheless, once in a while when I see a young, pregnant woman, I have this strange sadness that even if I wanted to, I wouldn't be able to get pregnant. I feel like a choice has been taken away from me.

♀ My best friend just told me about a friend of hers who got pregnant at 50 after not having a period for 5 years. 5 years! How is that even possible? This woman thought she was just gaining weight that she couldn't get rid of. She finally went to the doctor because she just couldn't control the weight gain. The doctor told her she was 6 months pregnant. She should be on one of those TV shows about amazing human anomalies. Can you even imagine what it must feel like to have a baby when you've already been an empty nester and thought you were post-menopausal? It scared me to death. My IUD is staying in until I am 60 just in case!

♀ Going through perimenopause was sort of like being pregnant. It seemed like everyone around you was going through the same thing. It also seemed like almost everything was affected by your physical condition. There were even times when I felt like it would have been kind of nice to have a lovely baby as a result, even though that isn't really what I wanted. I sort of felt physically like I did when I was pregnant. Now that I am post-menopausal, there is a tiny little sense of loss over not having the option of getting pregnant, but it is very, very tiny.

♀ I love this stage of life. My kids are grown, my husband and I have lots of time together, and I am starting to see a whole new phase of my life opening up. I am very happy that the mother-of-small-children phase is over. It was a very hard time that I loved, but wouldn't want to do again.

♀ I completely cracked up during the movie *Something's Gotta Give* when Jack Nicholson pauses just before having sex with Diane Keaton. He is used to having sex with much younger women, so even though she is much older than his typical partner, he is smart and asks, "Birth control?" She laughs and says, "Menopause!" His response is, "Lucky me!"

Lost and Found: Your Post-Menopausal Sense of Self

We can expect to be able to see our lives in a different way when the fluctuations, the wondering, and the periods are gone. In some cases, so we're told, women actually feel not only stable and functional again, but also experience a sense of dramatically increased accomplishment, energy, focus, and drive. It only seems fair! We contend that it isn't that post-menopausal women gain extra energy, focus, or drive. Instead, we propose that they just find what was lost during the perimenopausal stage!

Of course, there will still be adjustments to a new stage of life. However, while post-menopausal women may not feel like the same person they were before, they do tend to feel better about themselves, their relationships, and their lives.

♀ I actually feel younger and more energetic now that I am post-menopausal than I did during the years leading up to it.

♀ After menopause, I went from being a Type A person to a much more relaxed, slower-paced person. I kind of like it! There isn't as much stress and rushing in my life. I still get a lot done, but I'm not as worried.

♀ After menopause, I had the time and energy to do some of the things I had dreamed about doing for years. All the reasons for not doing them had gone away.

♀ After years of feeling tired and run down, I did get that spurt of energy that I've heard other women talk about. Now I just have to remember all those things I wanted to do. In the years leading up to menopause, I had lots of ideas, but no energy to follow through on any of them. Now I look back at some of them and think they were ridiculous, but there are a few that still have some merit. I feel so much better now that I am probably going to start taking action on the good ones. I hope my hubby can keep up with me!

♀ Throughout perimenopause, I felt like nothing I did was right. Even when something went well, I just didn't feel like I had met a worthwhile goal or accomplished something important. I think it was a combination of feeling like I was doing everything half-assed because I was so tired and moody and the fact that I didn't have a clear picture of what my life goals were. I may not have the big picture totally figured out now, but I don't feel like I need to. I have shorter-term goals that are achievable. I feel capable of making the decisions I need to make to get the things that are important to me. I am willing to invest my energy in the things I care about. Actually, one of the big differences is that I remember what I care about, when a few years ago, I didn't.

♀ I love looking at women in their 40's and early 50's and knowing that I already survived all the hard stuff they are going through now. It makes me feel strong, powerful, proud of myself, and really glad that period of my life is over!

♀ I am just now feeling like I am through all the drama of menopause. It took quite a while. I had my daughter when I was very young, so she is just now starting the process. I never talked about it when I was going through it, but now that she is discussing her experiences, I am opening up for the first time. I love that by talking about it I can help her know what to expect and get ideas for how to deal with it. When I hear myself talking about it, I feel really proud of myself for getting through it, too.

♀ My mother told me that she loved her 50's. She felt like she was past a lot of the turmoil in her life, she knew who she was, and she felt like herself again. When I was going through perimenopause, I constantly reminded myself that there was light at the end of the tunnel. It took me longer to get to that light that I had expected (and there were times when I was sure that light was a train coming towards me), but I did get there. I'm so glad my mom talked to me about it so I had something to look forward to when times were hard.

♀ I didn't really experience a lot of PMS until I was perimenopausal, when I could almost set my watch for a case of the blues to set in a few days before my period was due. I really hated that. I have been in "official" menopause for about a year now and am amazed at how much better I feel mentally, with minimal blue days and mood swings. The faucet still comes on over a good chick flick, though!

♀ It seemed like doctors, Web sites, my girlfriends, and my mother didn't really understand perimenopause, so it was hard to get good information and help a few years ago. Now that I am post-menopausal, it seems like there is much more helpful and consistent information about what is normal, what therapies are available, and what I can expect to have happen. It also seems like my doctor takes my concerns much more seriously. I sort of feel like I have graduated, so now I get some respect.

♀ I expect and strive to be happy, healthy, emotionally "present," and physically active despite any declines in vision, mental acuity, sexual

157

appetite, or anything else! What I don't want is to become a hateful, bitter, and mistrustful old biddy. So there!

♀ Back when I was having lots of hot flashes, huge unexpected periods, and uncontrollable appetite, osteoporosis was the least of my worries. I took calcium supplements, but had to deal with so many other things that were more bothersome. Now that I am post-menopausal, though, bone strength is one of my biggest concerns. I had adjusted to feeling older since I wasn't in the child-bearing years anymore, but worrying about getting a broken hip makes me feel positively ancient.

♀ After all the years of craziness, it took my husband a while to really believe that things had calmed down. He had heard so much about how hard menopause was that at first he kept expecting things to get worse after my periods completely stopped. Happily, it took a little while, but it became pretty clear that my moods and emotions had evened out and were pretty much staying that way.

♀ I survived perimenopause by making the conscious decision to be a true friend to my husband and not make him the scapegoat for my problems. I explained as best I could how I was feeling along the way, asked him for his support and help, and promised I wouldn't hurt him (and kept that promise even when it seemed impossible). I am so grateful that he believed me and we got through it.

♀ My husband and I have finally synced up with respect to sex. Neither of us wants it as much as we used to, but the amount seems right for both of us. We have finally established a new normal, which still includes using lubrication. He takes something to help him, which makes it better for both of us. All in all, this aspect of life isn't an issue now like it was a few years ago.

♀ I was single for most of my perimenopausal years. I hated my body so much that I couldn't imagine how anyone else would like it, so I was hesitant about getting seriously involved with anyone. Now I feel like I can trust my body not to embarrass me. Plus, most guys my age are a bit wrinkly and droopy, too, so they can't hold it against me unless they are the type of guy who wants a trophy wife on his arm. If that is what he wants, more power to him. He can go get it, and I won't be sad because that isn't the type of man I want anyway.

♀ During perimenopause, nothing in my life seemed right. I retired early, divorced my husband, and moved to a different town. I guess I thought that would get me what I wanted. So there I was, all alone in a new place with nothing to do, no more happy than I had been before. Over the next few years, as I moved into menopause, I became more able to differentiate between the things that were just irritating me and the things that were truly wrong. I started having a much clearer picture of what would make me happy. I finally had the energy to make some positive changes, rather than being sort of lazy and just dumping what I already had. I seriously wish I could go back in time and fix some of the mistakes I made when I was so hormonal, but all I can do now is be true to myself and make the best decisions I can at any given point in time.

♀ After years of feeling like I was lost, I feel like I have found myself again. It is a huge relief.

♀ The payoff from having symptoms like hot flashes and weight gain earlier in life than I expected is that things are better than I expected now that I am past menopause. Sure, I still sweat at times when other people are cold, but the mood swings and periods are gone. Happily, the constant questioning of myself and what my body is doing is also gone. I am much more content, much less stressed, and okay with being at the stage of life I'm at.

♀ The little stuff doesn't upset me so much these days. I realize how insignificant it is. I am not concerned with who likes me or how I look to someone. I can just be me and if I make connections with people, they are genuine and based on truth and not on appearances.

♀ My body, like everyone's, is constantly changing. I like to focus more on how I feel today and what I can accomplish rather than worrying about how my physical form is different from how it was when I was 25 or 30. I feel empowered and strong and am greatly appreciative of that. I take good care of myself with good nutrition, rest, and exercise. Also, the many beautiful people in my life fill me with gratitude, and as I grow older, I am aware of them so much more and, at the same time, aware of the energy vampires. Basically, despite some of the physical trade-offs (wrinkles, etc.), I am so energized at this time because of the wisdom I've gained through life experience. My relationship with my husband is better than ever. We have entered a new phase of our marriage – our kids are older and there is more time for us to be a couple. It is a wonderful and special time like we had when we were first married only better because we have more life experiences together.

♀ There are so many things that are better now. No more birth control hassles. I finally feel like my hormone level (or lack thereof) has stabilized so my moods have, too. I feel like myself in most ways. I like some new changes, like my ability to focus on myself without feeling guilty. Best of all, I can feel proud of myself for getting through the last 8 years of perimenopause without committing a violent crime, streaking naked through the streets, or locking myself in a padded room – all of which I felt like doing at one point or another before I finally reached menopause!

♀ Now that I am through menopause, I do feel "changed." I feel like I learned a lot from the experiences. Although I still do have occasional hot flashes and have vaginal dryness, I really like the woman I am today.

Conclusion

The Beginning of the Middle

We wish we could write about how we personally found a graceful way to survive the perimenopause years until, like butterflies, we emerged as happy, non-bleeding, calm, focused, energized, post-menopausal women who had found themselves again. Unfortunately, we are still in the midst of perimenopause and all its joys. We are better educated about the process, though. Best of all, we know that we are not alone. We are going through what millions of women have done before us, are doing with us, and will do after us. We are not imagining the heat, the leaking, the mental lapses, or the sense of disconnection of mind, body, and soul. Neither are you or the many women who shared their stories.

This is just our next stage of life. It is a roller coaster ride that is part of the journey that must be taken. We hope that we have encouraged you to acknowledge the ups and downs, navigate the twists and turns, grab onto good friends, and keep your eyes focused on the end of the ride so you can let go and laugh and scream your way through this very strange period.

Resources: Who Ya Gonna Call?

- www.astrangeperiod.com and http://facebook.com/astrangeperiod
- Jenny: 867-5309... jk =)
- The American College of Obstetricians and Gynecologists (including free online magazine): www.acog.org
- American Menopause Foundation: www.americanmenopause.org
- International Menopause Society/Council of Affiliated Menopause Societies: www.imsociety.org/cams
- Mayo Clinic: www.mayoclinic.com/health/perimenopause
- North American Menopause Society: www.menopause.org
- U.S. Department of Health and Human Services, The Office of Women's Health: www.womenshealth.gov/menopause
- Women to Women: www.womentowomen.com (We can't vouch for their services, but we like the information that is provided on the Web site and in their online newsletters)

Index: You Just Might Find, You Get What You Need

We recognize that indexes don't usually have introductory paragraphs; however, this one is a virtual crystal ball for the bizarre experience of perimenopause. Just reading through it will give you a pretty darn good overview of what to expect. Acne and aging and anal fissures, oh my!

About the Authors

Sheryl Gurrentz and Cindy Singer are BFFs who met when their oldest children were babies. In addition to working together in multiple companies, volunteering together on many non-profit fundraisers, inadvertently copying each others' clothes, jewelry, and furniture, and finishing each others' thoughts, they co-authored If Your Child is Bipolar. Sheryl is also the author of The Guilt-Free Guide to Your New Life as a Mom. Both books are National Parenting Publications Gold Parenting Resource Award winners. Sheryl has a degree in economics from the Wharton School of Business. Cindy has a degree in psychology from Colorado State University. The authors each have a wonderful husband and two kids. Both live in Denver, were born in early 1965, and started experiencing occasional mental lapses, strange periods, and embarrassing hair growth in their early 40's. Chances are, they both will finally emerge from perimenopause at about the same time and enter into the glory that certainly must follow. They hope it will be soon!

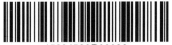

Made in the USA
Lexington, KY
25 May 2012